MW01291978

Martin Storr, MD

The FODMAP Compass

A Beginner`s Guide to the
Low-FODMAP Diet

Martin Storr, MD

The FODMAP Compass

A Beginner`s Guide to the
Low-FODMAP Diet

For People with Irritable Bowel Syndrome,
Wheat Intolerance and Other Digestive Disorders

1. English edition

 Zuckschwerdt Publishing, Munich

Thanks

Many thanks to Thierry Thirvaudey, the chef of the CIP Clinic Dr. Schlemmer in Bad Tölz, Bavaria, who cooked the recipes for this edition and arranged the dishes so wonderfully.

Title of the original german edition:

Der Ernährungsratgeber zur FODMAP-Diät – Die etwas andere Diät bei Reizdarm, Weizenunverträglichkeit und anderen Verdauungsstörungen (ISBN: 978-3-86371-206-8)

Cover design by W. Zuckschwerdt Verlag
© 2018 by W. Zuckschwerdt Verlag GmbH, Industriestraße 1, D-82110 Germering/München, Germany

Image index

© W. Zuckschwerdt Publishing House: Cover (FODMAP-letters) and all illustrations

© Fotolia: Cover tanjichica (Blueberries), P. 22 Marko Beckenbauer (Condensed Milk), P. 75 rainbow33 (Psyllium), P. 92 bit24 (Yogurt), P. 98 emuck (Dried fruits), P. 114 Jiri Hera (Maple Syrup), P. 121 mariontxa (Lemoncurd), P. 122 tashka2000 (Blueberry Pancake), P. 145 marysckin (Noodles), P. 158 kristina rütten (Bavarian Cream), P. 162 Quade (Banana)

© Shutterstock: P. 31 Ildi Papp (Pearjuice), P. 39 Edward Fielding (Lentils), P. 127 NADKI (Carrot/Turnip), P. 147 picturepartners (Pepper)

© Morguefile: P. 7, 12–13, 17, 21 (Onions, Peas), P. 23, 27, P. 31 (Apples), P. 35–37, P. 38 (Chickpeas), P. 39 (Sweets), P. 40–41, P. 8–9 and 52–53 (Cheese), P. 56, P. 59, P. 64–65, P. 76, P. 78–79, P. 94, P. 95–97, P. 99 (Onions), P. 101 (Quinoa), P. 105–106 (Flour), P. 110–111, P. 116–117, P. 120, P. 123–124, P. 127 (Mint), P. 127–131, P. 135, P. 138–139, P. 144, P. 146, P. 149–151, P. 154–155, P. 162–165, P. 168, P. 175

© All free Download: P. 17 (Peas), P. 20–21 (Wheat, Garlic), P. 22 (Chocolate), P. 16, P. 25 (Milk), P. 39 (Chewing Gum), P. 103 (Wheat, Tapioka), P. 125, S. 143 (Pepper)

Food-Photography © Felix Pitscheneder: P. 100, 113, 115, 119, 121, 137, 143, 153, 157, 161, 167, 173

Disclaimer:

The findings of medicine are subject to constant change through research and clinical experience. Author and publisher have taken great care to ensure that the information provided is up to date. However, this does not exempt the user of this book from the obligation to verify that the informations given here are factually correct. The book is not a substitute for medical advice and medical treatment.

The author and publisher disclaim, as far as the law allows, any liability arising directly or indirectly from the use, or misuse, of the information contained in this book.

All recipes have been formulated using ingredients known to be low-FODMAP at the time of publishing. While every effort has been taken to present low-FODMAP recipes, readers should assess their individual level of tolerance.

ISBN-13: 978-1721213993
ISBN-10: 1721213996

Preface

The organs involved in digestion work around the clock quietly and inconspicuously. When everything works perfectly, we do not notice anything except for the swallowing of food and the daily bowel movements. The consumed food passes through the esophagus, stomach, duodenum, the small intestine and the colon. It is digested during this passage. The share of it, which our body does not need, is ultimately excreted with the stool. Most of the time, we do not notice any of this. Only sometimes do we "feel" our digestive organs or hear one or the other sound coming from the belly.

But what if it does not work that smoothly? What happens when the intestine signals a problem manifested by stomach ache, bloating, diarrhea or constipation? Every gut has a bad day and not every intestinal rumbling is necessarily an indication of disease. But if the bad days become more frequent, if the bowel regularly gives off signals and the symptoms disturb the daily routine or impair the quality of life, then good advice should be sought.

The first thing to do is visit one's GP, who will try to get to the root cause. The mentioned symptoms may be a manifestation of a variety of diseases, from diarrhea caused by bacteria or viruses to constipation.

This Guide is not intended to replace any medical advice or treatment; hence, you should always first seek medical attention if you start experiencing symptoms, or if your symptoms change in the course of disease. In most cases, the altered bowel function is not caused by any serious disease. Very often, irritable bowel syndrome is diagnosed in connection with digestive complaints. Nearly 15 % of the German population have symptoms of irritable bowel syndrome or frequent digestive complaints. Nevertheless, most of them do not require any medical treatment, or require merely short-term therapy.

The low-FODMAP diet is based on the observation that some carbohydrates in our diet, called FODMAP carbohydrates, are not well-tolerated by all people and cause symptoms, especially in patients with a sensitive gut.

FODMAP carbohydrates are found in a wide variety of foods, and the low-FODMAP diet is not about healthy vs. unhealthy, but rather about well-digestible vs. poorly digestible. Numerous clinical trials have shown that a low-FODMAP diet is very effective in reducing digestive problems and may help patients with irritable bowel syndrome as well as other digestive disorders get their symptoms under control. Compared to drugs or probiotic therapy, the achievable therapeutic success is equivalent or even superior.

The aim of this Guide is to explain the rationale and effects of the low-FODMAP diet. With easy-to-use tips and delicious recipe suggestions, it will facilitate your transition to a low-FODMAP diet and thus to a future with as few digestive symptoms as possible.

I hope that you will enjoy reading this book as much as I enjoyed writing it. However, this Guide would never have seen the light of day in its present form without the invaluable suggestions of my wife and my mother. It was very much a joint effort.

Martin Storr, Munich, January 2018

Email of the author: FODMAP@gmx.de

Content

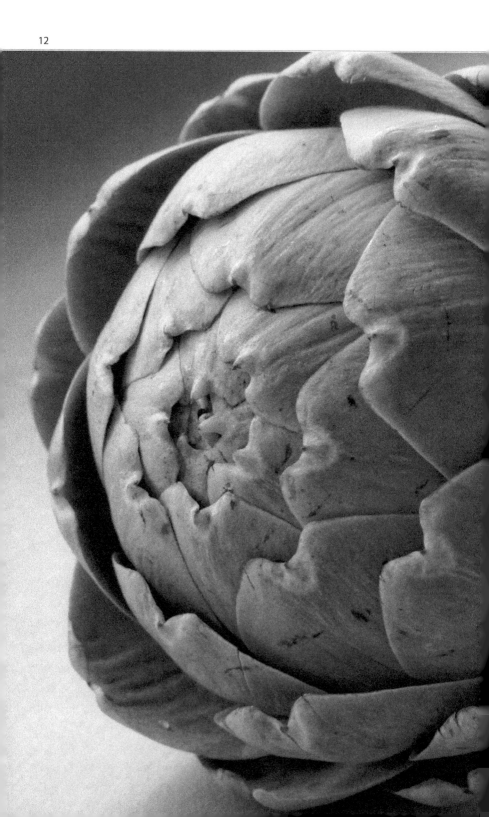

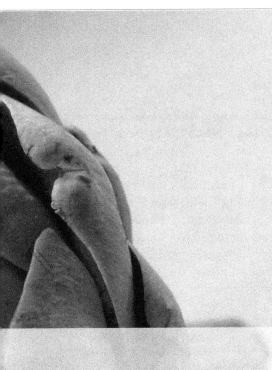

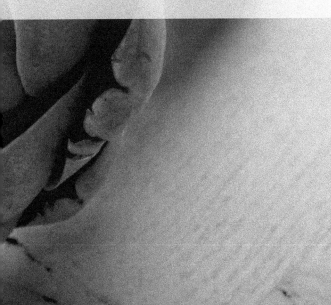

Chapter 1
FODMAPs

What is a FODMAP diet?

The FODMAP diet, or rather the low-FODMAP diet, is an elimination diet based on a novel dietary approach that has been specifically developed to prevent and/or treat digestive problems. Originally, the low-FODMAP diet was developed to provide relief from the symptoms of chronic inflammatory bowel disease (IBD) such as Crohn's disease and ulcerative colitis, as well as irritable bowel syndrome. However, it can also be used in other disorders manifesting with similar digestive symptoms like in functional GI disorders (FGID). The low-FODMAP diet effectively alleviates or prevents symptoms such as bloating, flatulence, abdominal pain, soft stools, frequent bowel movements, diarrhea and constipation.

 A low-FODMAP diet means consuming foods that are low in FODMAPs, while at the same time avoiding foods high in FODMAPs. This effectively reduces gastrointestinal complaints.

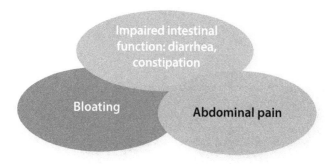

The low-FODMAP diet offers relief from intestinal complaints such as bloating, diarrhea, constipation and abdominal pain.

What are FODMAPs?

FODMAPs is an English acronym for fermentable oligosaccharides, disaccharides, monosaccharides and polyols.

FODMAPs are a collection of short-chain carbohydrates and sugar alcohols that are fermentable, meaning that they are broken down (fermented) in the large bowel (colon) by enzymes derived from bacteria. All nutrients summarized under the umbrella term "FODMAPs" are found in foods naturally or as food additives.

FODMAPs are not toxic or hazardous to health, but they can contribute to the development of gastrointestinal symptoms.

F	Fermentable	Fermentable
O	Oligosaccharides	multiple-unit sugars*
D	Disaccharides	double sugars
M	Monosaccharides	simple sugars
A	And	And
P	Polyols	Polyols

* Oligosaccharides consist of 3 to 10 monosaccharides

In 2005, a group of physicians and nutritionists from Australia hypothesized that the food, or more precisely the FODMAPs contained in the food, are responsible for the development and aggravation of GI symptoms in patients with inflammatory bowel disease. This hypothesis was based on their own observations as well as on the analysis of numerous nutritional protocols of patients with inflammatory bowel disease. These nutritional protocols revealed that the patients had consumed an excess of foods high in FODMAPs, and this observation formed the basis for the FODMAP hypothesis.

FODMAPs are a broad variety of food ingredients. From a digestive viewpoint, FODMAPs have three main characteristics in common:

Absorption in the small intestine is difficult or impossible

FODMAPs are poorly or not at all absorbed in the small intestine. The reasons include the following:

- ▶ Some molecules such as polyols (sugar alcohols) are too large to pass through the intestinal wall;
- ▶ The transport capacities through the intestinal wall are limited, as is the case with fructose (fructose malabsorption);
- ▶ The enzyme activity facilitating the transport through the intestinal wall is deficient, as is the case with lactose and its corresponding enzyme lactase;
- ▶ The small intestine lacks the corresponding enzymes to hydrolyze breakdown into digestible components, as is the case with fructans (fructo-oligosaccharides) and galactans (galacto-oligosaccharides).

High water-binding capacity

In technical terms, FODMAPs are said to have a very high water-binding capacity. FODMAPs are small molecules which can bind a large amount of water. This causes fluid to accumulate in the intestine and in turn leads to an increased transport speed in the intestine with frequent bowel movements and softer stools, including diarrhea.

Rapid fermentation by gut bacteria

All FODMAPs are rapidly fermented by bacteria resident in the gut. The exact rate of bacterial fermentation depends on the length of the carbohydrate chains. FODMAPs are all short-chained and hence rapidly fermented. As a result, they trigger symptoms rather quickly.

Are all carbohydrates FODMAPs?

Carbohydrates come in a variety of forms in foods, namely as simple carbohydrates, which include monosaccharides (simple sugars) such as glucose and fructose and disaccharides (double sugars) such as sucrose and lactose, as well as complex carbohydrates (polysaccharides).

The latter are further subdivided into short-chain and long-chain polysaccharides. Long-chain polysaccharides, in turn, include digestible starch and non-digestible polysaccharides such as cellulose, the structural component of the primary cell wall of green plants.

Carbohydrates are an important part of our diet. Most FODMAPs are carbohydrates, but not all carbohydrates are FODMAPs. FODMAP-carbohydrates are a well-defined group of short-chain carbohydrates.

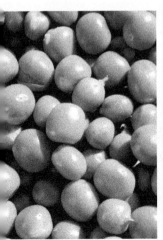 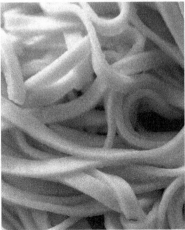 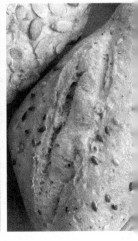

Most foods high in FODMAPs contain short-chain carbohydrates, which are poorly absorbed in the small intestine.

How do FODMAPs cause symptoms?

FODMAPs are short-chain carbohydrates and sugar alcohols, which are moderately to scarcely digestible and therefore reach the colon via the small intestine in a nearly undigested form. In the colon, FODMAPs are subsequently fermented by the intestinal bacteria, also called intestinal flora. FODMAPs are decomposed during fermentation. This produces energy and various degradation products, including many gases such as hydrogen. These gases that accumulate in the intestine cause symptoms, especially bloating and flatulence. Both symptoms are reported very frequently by patients with irritable bowel syndrome, but also by those with other GI disorders.

Since FODMAPs are inevitably a part of any balanced diet, the FODMAP theory assumes that patients who develop digestive complaints display specific characteristics: On the one hand, the ingestion of FODMAPs with food intake is increased; on the other hand, however, the small intestine of these patients can absorb less FODMAPs. These two causes can be present separately or in combination, with the inevitable consequence of a higher amount of FODMAPs reaching the colon.

What makes the FODMAP concept revolutionary?

The fact that individual FODMAPs such as lactose, fructose or sweeteners cause symptoms is not new knowledge. For decades, we have been aware of the resulting symptoms of diarrhea and bloating. In the past, individual diets with a reduced content of lactose, fructose or gluten have been described as possibly helpful for patients with irritable bowel syndrome. All these diets assume that one or more food ingredients are responsible for the symptoms, and that the symptoms improve when fewer of these food ingredients are ingested. However, all these diets have proven inefficient or – at best – minimally efficient in reducing the symptoms in patients suffering from irritable bowel syndrome.

The revolutionary aspect of the FODMAP concept is that a single diet now captures all these small molecules rather than individual ones. The objective of this diet is not to completely eliminate all FODMAPs, but rather the concept proposes to control and reduce the amount of FODMAPs as much as possible. The goal is to reduce the total amount of FODMAPs in the food we consume to such an extent that the remaining FODMAPs no longer cause any symptoms.

 A low-FODMAP diet does not eliminate solely individual substances that may cause GI complaints; rather, it reduces all substances causing symptoms. The goal is to significantly reduce the total amount of FODMAPs.

The FODMAP theory does not mean to suggest that FODMAPs are a root cause of diseases. Irritable bowel syndrome and chronic inflammatory bowel diseases have other causes – it is not due to the FODMAP content in our food. Rather, the FODMAP theory assumes that FODMAPs are involved in the development of symptoms, particularly in the case of an existing disease and in the case of existing digestive complaints, i.e. the annoying bloating, soft stools, diarrhea and intestinal cramps.

Therefore, the goal of a low-FODMAP diet is not to treat the root cause of irritable bowel syndrome, but rather to offer a way of eventually reducing and/or avoiding symptoms. This is highly relevant and progressive as previous IBS diets were always tailored around the presumed pathological digestion or intolerances, such as lactose or fructose intolerance.

FODMAPs are present in the food we consume and they are delivered to the colon – that is completely normal. It is also normal that these FODMAPs are fermented in the colon by bacteria. Gastrointestinal symptoms, however, are effectively reduced if the absolute quantity of FODMAPs entering the colon is reduced by means of a consistent dietary change.

Which substances are grouped under the umbrella term 'FODMAPs'?

The term 'FODMAPs' encompasses fermentable oligosaccharides, disaccharides and monosaccharides as well as polyols. FODMAPs are contained in almost all foodstuffs, and you will learn more about individual FODMAPs and the FODMAP content of different foods. The first step is to become familiar with FODMAPs and to understand which FODMAPs are contained in various foodstuffs. Later, you will learn how this concept can be translated into a relevant diet.

The terms oligosaccharides, disaccharides, monosaccharides and polyols do not mean much to most people. We do not automatically associate any food ingredients with these terms. Therefore, it is important to recognize to what specific food ingredients these terms refer.

The terms oligosaccharides, disaccharides and monosaccharides refer to multiple-unit sugars, double sugars and simple sugars, respectively. The table shows which substances belong to the individual groups, and which foods contain them.

FODMAPs: An Overview

Group	Appear in the diet as ...	Are abundantly contained in ...
Oligosaccharides	Fructans Galactans Fructo-oligosaccharides (FOS) Galacto-oligosaccharides (GOS)	Barley, rye, wheat, peas, garlic, leeks, lentils, onions
Disaccharides	Lactose	Yogurt, milk, cream
Monosaccharides	Fructose	Apples, pears, honey, cherries, corn sirup, asparagus
Polyols	Sorbitol (Sorbit) Mannitol (Mannit) Maltitol (Maltit) Xylitol (Xylit)	Apples, pears, cherries, nectarines, plums, diet products, chewing gum, sweeteners

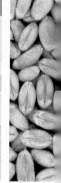

Oligosaccharides

Oligosaccharides are various sugars composed of at least three sugar molecules. All oligosaccharides are therefore carbohydrates.

Depending on how many monosaccharides the oligosaccharides are composed of, they are referred to as

- Trisaccharides (three molecules of monosaccharides),
- Tetrasaccharides (four molecules of monosaccharides), or
- Pentasaccharides (five molecules of monosaccharides).

This designation based on the exact number could be continued. It is, however, unusual to use this exact counting method.

For simplification purposes, the term oligosaccharides is often used for sugars consisting of 3 to 10 monosaccharides. Longer carbohydrate chains, i.e. those containing more than 10 aligned monosaccharides, are called polysaccharides (multiple-unit sugars), and they play no role in the FODMAP diet.

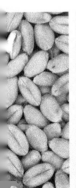
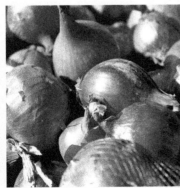
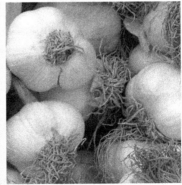
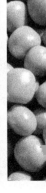

Fructans, galactans and galacto-oligosaccharides are oligosaccharides (multiple-unit sugars) that are relevant for the FODMAP concept. Fructans, which also include fructo-oligosaccharides (FOS), are short-chain carbohydrates consisting of very short chains of several fructose molecules and a glucose molecule at the end of the chain. Galactans are short branched-chain carbohydrates composed of individual galactose molecules. Galacto-oligosaccharides (GOS), on the other hand, are short-chain carbohydrates with chains of several galactose molecules and a glucose molecule at the end of the chain. All these oligosaccharides occur naturally and are standard food components.

Disaccharides

'Disaccharide' is the technical term for a double sugar. There are numerous disaccharides which we take in with food and which are well-digested by our intestines or insignificant for symptom generation and therefore do not play any role in the FODMAP diet. The table lists various disaccharides that are ingested with food, of which lactose is relevant for the FODMAP diet.

Disaccharides (double sugars)

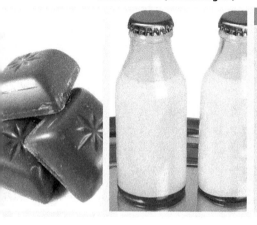

FODMAP-reich	FODMAP-arm
Lactose	Cellobiose
	Gentobiose
	Isomaltose
	Kojibiose
	Maltose
	Nigerose
	Primverose
	Rutinose
	Sucrose
	Trehalose

Monosaccharides

Monosaccharides are simple sugars. Simple sugars act as energy carriers in foods and are formed in a myriad of variations in our metabolism. The simple sugar fructose is the only sugar from the group of monosaccharides that is relevant for the FODMAP diet. Other simple sugars that we take in with foodstuffs such as glucose, galactose, mannose, xylose and arabinose play no role in the FODMAP diet.

Polyols

From a chemical perspective, polyols are polyhydric alcohols. These alcohols are present in natural foodstuffs in various forms. Polyols occur naturally in a wide variety of fruits and vegetables, and provide the taste and texture of sugar with about half the calories.

Due to their sweet taste, these polyols are very often used by the food industry as sugar substitutes. Sorbitol, mannitol and xylitol, as well as the names of many other polyols or their corresponding European EXXX numbers for the labeling of food additives, can be found in the list of ingredients of many foodstuffs. For a detailed listing of polyols

Natural foods containing polyols

Sorbitol	Mannitol
Apple	Mushrooms
Apricot	Seaweed
Peach	
Pear	
Plum	
Large amounts in dried fruits	

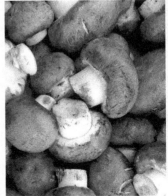
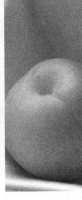

and food additive names, please refer to the table on page 39. You will be surprised by the widespread presence of polyols in our foods, as well as in other products such as toothpaste or mouthwash. Due to the desire for a calorie-reduced nutrition, the proportion of polyols in our diet is increasing exponentially.

Frequently occuring FODMAPs

The list of FODMAPs contains some well-known food ingredients occurring regularly and in large quantities in our food, such as lactose (milk sugar), fructose (fruit sugar), variations of fructose such as fructans and galacto-oligosaccharides, and some polyols.

Since these are food ingredients that are present in our usual diet, and quite notably in a healthy diet, it is a good idea to examine these food components more closely. This will help you recognize what to look for and how to shape your future diet.

Lactose content in dairy products

Very high in lactose	High in lactose	Moderate lactose content	Hardly any lactose
More than 10 g/100 g	4–10 g/100 g	1–4 g/100 g	Less than 1 g/100 g
Condensed milk Creamer	Buttermilk	Cottage cheese	Brie cheese
Milk powder	Coffee creamer	Cream cheese	Butter
Whey cheese	Ice cream	Curd	Camembert cheese
Whey powder	Skimmed milk	Kefir	Feta cheese
	Milk chocolate	Low-fat curd	Hard cheese
	Whey	Nut-nougat cream	
	Whole milk	Sour Cream	
		Whipped cream	
		Yogurt	

Lactose

Also referred to as "milk sugar," lactose is a disaccharide, composed of the monosaccharide components glucose and galactose. In our intestine, the enzyme lactase breaks down lactose into two monosaccharides. Only after this decomposition can the two monosaccharide components be absorbed into the bloodstream through the intestinal wall and used as energy carriers. Humans are born naturally able to produce ample amounts of lactase in order to digest mother's milk that is very rich in lactose while nursing.

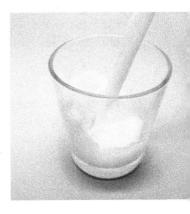

Lactase activity in the intestine decreases with age since we do not feed on mother's milk for a lifetime, and the consumption of milk and dairy products decreases with advancing age.

In regions like Europe where dairy products are consumed for a lifetime, there is higher intestinal lactase activity in adults than in regions where dairy products are not consumed, such as in Africa or Southeast Asia. In western societies, approximately two-thirds of adults still have measurable intestinal lactase activity, while the remaining one-third have no measurable lactase activity. The figures below show the extent of this distinctive geographic distribution of lactase activity in adults. While 98 % of adults in the Scandinavian countries have a detectable intestinal lactase activity, only less than 10 % of adults in Africa or Asia have a measurable lactase activity. For most people, the intestinal lactase activity is irrelevant, since the diet in the adult age is no longer based exclusively on dairy products. Rather, it includes merely low amounts of dairy products.

Precisely because our diet contains little lactose, a diminished or an altogether absent lactase activity in the intestine is insignificant for most people in the adult age.

Lactose, which is not broken down in the small intestine because there is insufficient enzyme or enzyme activity, cannot be absorbed into the bloodstream from the intestine. Unchanged, the lactose enters the colon where it is then fermented by colonic bacteria, giving rise to bacterial degradation products, including many gases which in turn can cause discomfort.

For this reason, the lack of lactase activity is revealed in some adults when they get GI complaints, especially when their diet contains many dairy products. A diet that is rich in dairy products is generally not unhealthy if one tolerates it well. The symptoms caused by lactose can range from occasional mild symptoms to frequent and severe symptoms.

In the case of frequent symptoms that seem to be induced by lactose, a physician should be consulted to check for lactose intolerance. If confirmed, special dietary recommendations should be considered.

 When eating foods high in lactose induces symptoms on a regular basis, a physician should be consulted to check for lactose intolerance.

What foods contain lactose?

The "milk sugar" lactose is contained in all dairy products such as milk, cheese, yogurt and curd. Normal cow's milk, for example, contains between 4 and 8 % lactose. The exact lactose content varies depending on the origin of the milk; cow's milk, for example, has a different lactose content than sheep milk, goat milk or horse milk. Lactose is found in all dairy products, but in varying amounts depending on how the dairy product has been further processed. The table on page 24 shows the lactose content of different dairy products.

A lesser-known but interesting fact is that lactose is often added as a stabilizer or flavoring agent in industrially processed foods. Therefore, you should always read the list of ingredients of processed foods carefully to see where lactose has been added. Furthermore, lactose is found in numerous medications as a diluent or filler, since lactose is very cost effective and inherently compactable, that is, able to form a solid compact (i.e. tablet) under compression. However, the lactose content of medicinal products should not be taken into account due to the very small amounts.

Fructose

Fructose is a simple sugar with a very high sweetness level. It is found naturally in herbal products. Foods naturally rich in fructose include honey, raisins and other dried fruits. Fructose is extracted from sugar cane, sugar beet or corn. In addition to glucose, all three plants contain high amounts of fructose. Owing to its high sweetness level, simple extraction and, in some cases also due to its brown color, fructose is often added to food and beverages. Information on the fructose content of each food is indicated in the list of ingredients.

There are several reasons why fructose is poorly or not at all absorbed in the small intestine. It may be that too much fructose is contained in the food, the food is transported too rapidly through the small intestine, or that the number of the intestinal fructose transporters (GLUT-5) is too low or their activity too weak.

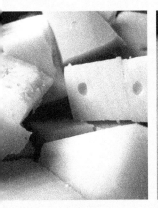
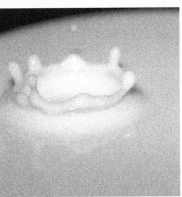
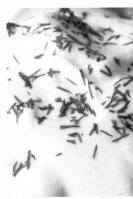

Lactose is found in varying amounts in all dairy products. It is also used as a stabilizer and flavoring agent in other foods.

When eating foods high in fructose induces symptoms on a regular basis, a physician should be consulted to check for fructose malabsorption.

Breath hydrogen testing can be used to detect malabsorption of fructose, i.e. a restricted fructose uptake. Alternative terms for fructose malabsorption are dietary fructose intolerance or intestinal fructose intolerance

A completely different disease is hereditary fructose intolerance, a very rare hereditary metabolic disease. This disease is detected by genetic testing. Due to all these various terms, one must carefully consider which disorder is exactly meant.

Ways of fructose absorption

Since fructose is a simple sugar, it does not have to be broken down in the intestine before it can be absorbed into the bloodstream. It is first taken as a whole from the intestine by the intestinal absorptive cells (enterocytes) and then released from them into the bloodstream. This uptake and release of fructose by the enterocytes is regulated by a special transport protein located in the cell walls. The transport protein for fructose is named GLUT-5.

Usually, fructose is completely absorbed across the intestine into the bloodstream. Fructose digestion becomes a problem only when there is too much fructose in the intestine. In such a case, the absorptive capacity of the body may become exhausted and the transport function of GLUT-5 overloaded. As a consequence, fructose is incompletely absorbed into the bloodstream from the small intestine and it enters the colon.

 For various reasons, modern-day diets can contain very high amounts of fructose. In a normal, balanced diet, fructose content often exceeds the absorptive capacity of our bodies.

The intestine can absorb approximately 35–50 g of fructose per day using the fructose transporter. The average daily amount of consumed fructose (50–60 g) already slightly exceeds the normal uptake capacity of a human being. Since these figures indicate the average intake, it is very clear that in many people the fructose intake with their diet significantly exceeds the uptake capacity of the intestine.

However, fructose uptake from the intestine into the body is subject to a few additional properties. For one, the fructose transporter Glut-5 can be blocked by polyols like sorbitol. Therefore, a diet rich in sorbitol (e.g. consuming sorbitol-rich plums) results in a diminished fructose uptake in the intestine. Furthermore, diseases such as hypertension, diabetes and obesity can diminish fructose uptake, because these diseases are associated by an impaired activity of the fructose transporter.

It is exactly the opposite in the presence of glucose. The presence of glucose in the intestine facilitates the uptake of fructose. That is why fruit containing a balanced ratio of fructose and glucose is better digestible than fruit that is naturally rich in fructose.

What happens to fructose in the colon?

Fructose, which is not absorbed in the small intestine, enters the colon where it is fermented by the intestinal bacteria or fungi (yeasts). This results in bacterial degradation products and gases such as carbon dioxide, which can cause discomfort. In contrast to the long-chain fructans and galactans, the fermentation of fructose is faster, meaning that the intake of fructose leads to symptoms more rapidly.

What makes fructose so attractive to food processing industry?

There are several reasons why fructose is often used in industrially processed foods. One reason is certainly the high sweetness value of fructose. Compared to glucose, fructose is two and a half times sweeter. This difference is even greater when compared to lactose – fructose is eleven times sweeter than lactose. In view of this, it is easy to understand why fructose is the preferred agent in industrial food processing.

However, there are other reasons for the use of fructose. Sometimes, fructose is used in industrial food processing since it can form chemical compounds with the proteins contained in the foods. The advantage of these compounds is the formation of a light brownish discoloration; hence, in this context, fructose can be referred to as a sweetener and food coloring agent. Fructose is used as a food coloring agent when a light brown color of the resulting product is desired such as in bread and other pastries. Furthermore, fructose is used in beverage production. Yeasts used in the production of alcoholic beverages can ferment fructose as well as glucose. Such fructose-containing drinks have a slightly higher residual sweetness and are also suitable for diabetics in limited amounts. The desired end-products are alcohol and carbon dioxide, which initially remains dissolved in the beverage and is released only upon opening the bottle.

What is the significance of the ratio of glucose to fructose?

In connection with the fructose content of fruits, the sucrose content of these foods is also important, since the disaccharide sucrose is broken down into the simple sugars glucose and fructose. For this reason, sucrose too has to be regarded as a source of fructose.

The glucose-to-fructose ratio in foods plays a very significant role in the assessment of their tolerability. A ratio greater than 1 (> 1) implies more glucose than fructose and hence a better tolerability. Some examples can be found in the table on page 33.

A ratio less than 1 (< 1) implies more fructose than glucose and hence a poorer tolerability.

On the whole, however, the glucose-to-fructose ratio plays a less significant role than the absolute fructose content.

Fruits contain fructose and sucrose in different amounts. Apples and pears, for example, are extremely rich in fructose, while apricots and peaches are low in fructose.

Fructose is also contained in products which we do not immediately associate with the term fructose, such as honey or molasses, i.e. sugar beet sirup. Both are products that can be consumed on their own as spreads, or as additions to other foods (sweeteners). Corn syrup, for instance, is very complex when it comes to considering its fructose content. It is frequently found in the list of ingredients of foods and is used as a sweetener. In its inherent form, corn syrup consists main-

Foods high in fructose content

Dried fruits	Apple	
	Date	
	Mango	
	Pear	
	Raisins/sultanas	
Obst frisch	Apple	
	Cherry	
	Fig	
	Mango	
	Pear	
	Persimmon (kaki)	
Cerealien	Crunchy honey flakes	
	Honeygranola/muesli	
Other foods	Fruit concentrates	
	Fruit juice	
	Honey	
	Instant beverages	
	Invert sugar sirup	
	Products for diabetics	

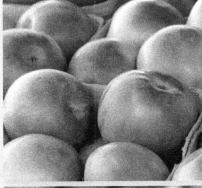
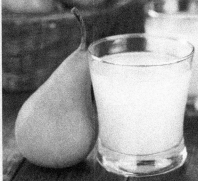

ly of glucose. In food processing industry, however, it can be treated enzymatically, so that the glucose contained in it is converted into fructose. Such enzymatically-treated corn syrup is referred to as glucose-fructose syrup (the German term) or high-fructose corn syrup (HFCS) (the English term). This enzymatic conversion is advantageous since fructose has a higher sweetening level at the same sugar quantity. The fructose content in corn syrup can be increased to a maximum of 90 %.

The European Union Sugar Directive from 2001 states that any sugar sirup with at least a 5 % fructose content must be declared as a glucose-fructose syrup or fructose-glucose syrup.

Is an increased fructose content in the diet damaging to health?

In small quantities, fructose is not unhealthy as it is a naturally-occurring sugar. Neither a carcinogenic nor a mutagenic effect of fructose has been reported thus far.

However, the consumption of fructose is nevertheless associated with some risks. Glucose is absorbed by the body and then consumed or stored in the metabolism under the control of the body's hormone insulin.

Fructose is also absorbed from the intestine into the bloodstream and reaches the liver where it is introduced into the body's metabolism, independently of the body's insulin, i.e. in a somewhat uncontrolled manner. Therefore, fructose is said to have negative effects on our health, especially when the fructose intake is very high. Excessive fructose consumption is presumably a cause of obesity (an excessive weight gain), fatty liver disease, the dangerous insulin resistance (a precursor to diabetes), as well as of the metabolic syndrome and disorders of lipid metabolism. Furthermore, it is assumed that fructose does not induce a feeling of satiety to the same extent as glucose does, a further mechanism that leads to an increased hunger sensation and ultimately to weight gain.

Glucose-fructose ratio of selected fruits and honey

Fruit	Glucose	Fructose	Ratio	
	Grams per 100 g		< 0,5	0,5–1
Apple	2,0	5,7	0,4	
Apple dried	9,8	27,8	0,4	
Blueberry	2,5	3,3		0,7
Currant	2,0	2,5		0,8
Gooseberry	3,0	3,3		0,9
Kiwi	4,3	4,6		1,0
Mango	0,9	2,6	0,3	
Orange	2,3	2,6		0,9
Peach	1,0	1,2		0,8
Pear	1,7	6,7	0,2	
Pineapple	2,1	2,4		0,9
Raspberry	1,8	2,1		0,8
Strawberry	2,2	2,2		1,0
Watermelon	2,0	3,9		0,5
Honey	33,9	38,8		0,9

There are significant gaps in our current understanding of fructose and much remains speculative at the moment. There are, however, very clear indications from medical research that our bodies cannot handle fructose as well as glucose.

This should not be a problem for people who eat normally, that is to say for those who do not consume excessive amounts and have no malabsorption issues. The unfavorable metabolic properties of fructose become problematic only when the fructose content in the diet increases too much, as is currently the case.

Why is the fructose content in our diet increasing?

The answers to the previous questions have already indicated that fructose offers advantages over glucose in industrial food processing and is therefore increasingly contained in our foods in terms of quantity and spectrum of foods.

However, this is not the only reason why the fructose content in our diet is steadily increasing. Another reason is that our diet should be increasingly healthy and we are supposed to eat healthier foods. But much of what appears healthy at first sight is, when studied closely, not as healthy as we thought.

For instance, a fruit bar has a much higher fructose content than the consumption of the comparable quantity of fresh fruit. Another very clear example is that a glass of apple juice, which contains the best of four apples, naturally also contains the fructose quantity of four apples.

The fructose content in our diet has increased exponentially. In some people, the gastrointestinal tract cannot cope with this excess supply of fructose, resulting in symptoms.

In many people, the gastrointestinal tract handles it well, but in some people, the gastrointestinal tract cannot cope with this excess supply of fructose, and symptoms develop, particularly when the intestine is additionally overloaded with an excess of other FODMAPs.

To what extent is fructose consumption increasing?

For the European population, there are currently no good figures on the average daily fructose consumption. Old estimates predict that an adult in central Europe will take in an average of 50–60 g of fructose per day. This corresponds to approximately 20 kg of fructose per year.

There are far better estimates on the sugar consumption of refined (i..e. industrially processed) sugar in the United States of America. The total sugar consumption has risen from 40 kg of sugar per capita

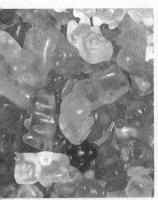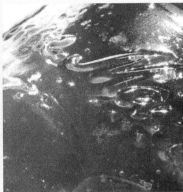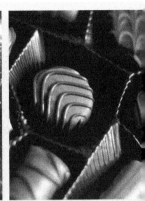

The consumption of refined fructose has risen strongly with the consumption of industrially processed foods.

per year in the seventies of the last century to a current 50 kg of refined sugar. It is interesting to note that the consumption of refined fructose was less than 1 kg per capita per year in the seventies, while now it is as high as 20 kg per capita per year. This amount of refined fructose is consumed via the industrially processed foods in addition to our consumption of natural fructose. From these numbers it becomes clear that the strong rise in fructose in our diet is caused primarily by the industrially processed foodstuffs.

Fructans

Fructans (fructo-oligosaccharides/FOS and fructo-polysaccharides) are multi-unit sugars consisting of a glucose ring and at least two fructose rings. Fructans with less than ten fructose rings are called fructo-oligosaccharides, and fructans with more than ten fructose rings are called inulins. In addition to starch and sucrose, fructans are the most important herbal carbohydrate stores. In addition to plants, some bacteria and yeasts can also produce and store fructans.

Fructans occur naturally in a variety of foods such as, characteristically, onions which are high in fructans. Substantial quantities of fructans are also found in cereals, beetroot, tubers and sprouts. A very high content of fructans is also found in topinambur tubers and chicory roots. The fructan content varies depending on the cultivation conditions such as season, temperature and precipitation.

The names of fructans are hardly known; on occasion, the terms 'levans' and 'inulins' are found on food packaging. The table on the next page shows a list of foods high in fructans.

Chicory is very interesting as it is used not only as a salad, but also for the production of coffee, or, more precisely, substitute coffee. This substitute coffee is known as 'country coffee', 'chicory root coffee' or 'carob coffee', as well as 'chicory water' in Austria.

What happens to fructans in the intestine?

The human small intestine does not produce enzymes capable of hydrolyzing fructans, and as such they cannot be absorbed across the small intestine. Therefore, they are delivered to the large bowel. Due to their indigestibility, fructans are used to a small extent as additives for dietary and diabetic products. Therefore, fructans are often listed in the lists of ingredients of these products. Fructans are used as additives as they are considered calorie-free dietary fiber.

These added fructans are to be considered for a FODMAP diet. On average, we consume about 10 g of fructans daily. The human body can handle this amount well. They are broken down by the colonic

Foods high in fructans

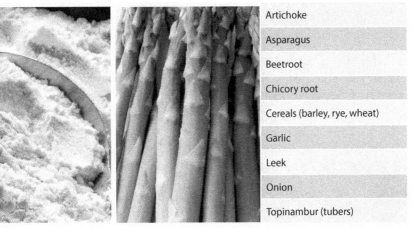

Artichoke
Asparagus
Beetroot
Chicory root
Cereals (barley, rye, wheat)
Garlic
Leek
Onion
Topinambur (tubers)

bacteria, and various degradation products, especially gases, develop, just as in the case of lactose and fructose entering the colon. Since fructans may be both short-chained or long-chained, some fructans are associated with a more rapid development of symptoms than others.

Galactans and galacto-oligosaccharides

Galactans and galacto-oligosaccharides are carbohydrates consisting of several sugar rings. Galacto-oligosaccharides are simple chains of up to eight sugar rings, while galactans are branched chains. At least one of these sugar rings is the simple sugar galactose, from which galactans got their name.

Galacto-oligosaccharides are natural ingredients of numerous foods. Typical galacto-oligosaccharides are raffinose, a triple-unit sugar consisting of fructose, glucose and galactose, and stachyose, a four-unit sugar consisting of fructose, glucose and two galactose rings. Large amounts of these galacto-oligosaccharides are found in legumes such as beans, lentils and soybean. Galactans occur naturally mainly in the plant cell walls. Because of their gel-forming properties, galactans are frequently used in food processing as thickening or gelling agents. Frequently used galactans are carrageenans from algae (E 407), agar agar (E 406) and tragacanth, a natural polysaccharide produced from the tree Astralagus gummifer (E 413).

Like other FODMAPs, galacto-oligosaccharides and galactans cannot be absorbed or digested in our intestine since the available enzymes cannot hydrolyze the bonds between the sugar rings in these chains.

Foods high in galacto-oligosaccharides and galactans

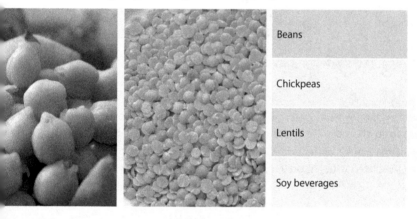

Beans

Chickpeas

Lentils

Soy beverages

Natural and synthetic polyols

Sugar alcohols, or polyols, are a group of ingredients that are used as sugar substitutes in our diet. The most well-known polyols are mannitol and sorbitol.

The name designation is in some cases somewhat confusing i.e. sorbitol is also known as hexanhexol or glucitol. For all other polyolstheir names usually end with –ol like mannitol or xylitol. These sugar substitutes are mostly produced synthetically and in the European Union they are additionally labeled with an E number for food additives (E XXX). You will find a list of polyols below.

In North America, many foods such as sweets and, in particular, chewing gum, are often labeled with health warnings, which indicate that polyols contained may cause diarrhea, as gum addicts will readily confirm.

Polyols also occur naturally. A relatively large amount of sorbitol is for example found in apples, pears, plums and peaches. Polyols are hardly metabolized in the small intestine or absorbed across the small intestine and are thus delivered to the colon in an undigested form. Like other FODMAPs, they too are fermented by colonic bacteria.

Polyols and their E numbers for food additive labeling

Name	E-number
Erythritol	E 968
Isomaltol	E 953
Lactitol	E 966
Maltitol	E 965
Mannitol	E 421
Sorbitol, Sorbit	E 420
Xylitol, Xylit	E 967

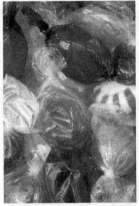
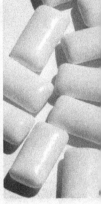

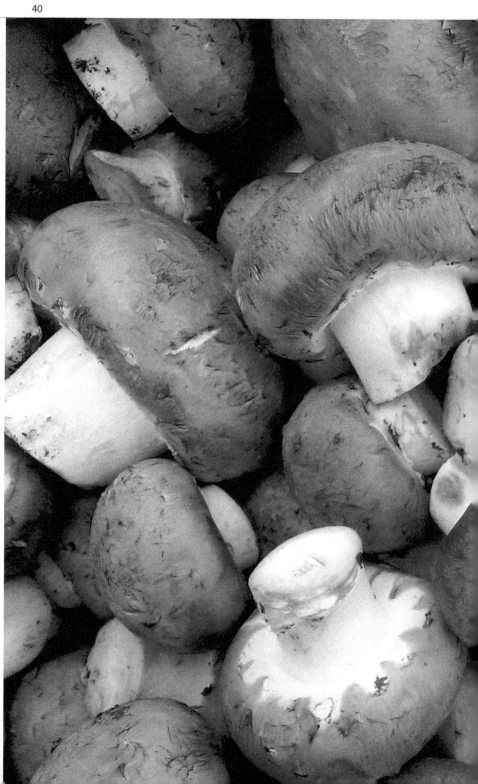

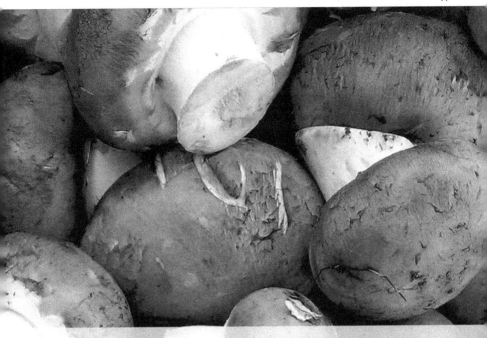

Chapter 2
When do FODMAPs become a problem?

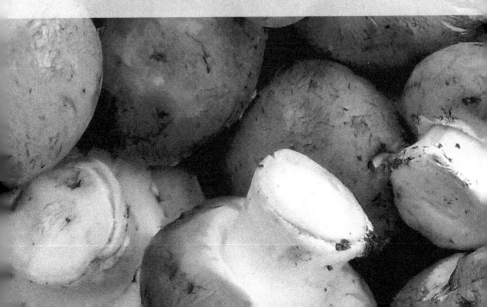

What symptoms do FODMAPs cause?

FODMAPs, or rather an excess of FODMAPs, mainly cause digestive problems. Various studies revealed that a diet high in FODMAPs can worsen symptoms, while a diet low in FODMAPs alleviates symptoms. Digestive symptoms aggravated by FODMAPs include bloating, flatulence, abdominal pain, diarrhea, constipation, heartburn, and nausea.

Interestingly, several studies showed that even fatigue, decreased drive, lethargy, and a poor mood improved when switching to a low-FODMAP diet. This is most likely due to the fact that digestive problems affect the entire body. Noteworthily, the improvements achieved by a low-FODMAP diet are at least as good as the improvements brought about by medications or probiotic treatments.

> An excess in FODMAPs leads to digestive symptoms, most notably to bloating, flatulence, abdominal pain, diarrhea, constipation and heartburn, but also to fatigue and lethargy.

Does everyone get symptoms from FODMAPs?

No. Although FODMAPs are poorly digested by all people – the healthy and patients with digestive problems alike – not all people develop symptoms. Symptoms tend to occur only in some people, more precisely in those with a particularly sensitive and susceptible gut.

The line here is rather fuzzy, which means that healthy people too can occasionally experience flatulence, increased intestinal gas, or loose stools. If this occurs only occasionally, it is not really a problem. There's more than a grain of truth in the well-known sentence „Every little bean will make its own little sound" (referring to flatulence related to consumption of legumes).

Why do FODMAPs cause symptoms in some people?

The reasons why some people experience symptoms after consuming FODMAPs include:

- ► intestinal hypersensitivity, i.e. a sensitive gut;
- ► a change in the activity of the intestinal muscles and hence a modified transport speed, and
- ► a change in the composition of the bacteria resident in the intestine with the resulting modification of gas formation caused by FODMAPs.

What happens with FODMAPs in the small intestine?

In the small intestine, FODMAPs are neither digested nor absorbed, but rather they are transported directly into the colon in an unchanged form. During this transport, FODMAPs bind water in the small intestine. This water binding is called osmotic activity. The increased water bound in the intestine contributes to diarrhea, while the increased formation of gas in the small intestine causes abdominal pain since the small intestine is particularly sensitive.

In addition, it is believed that small intestinal bacterial overgrowth and altered intestinal microbiota is a feature in irritable bowel syndrome (IBS) patients. This colonization of the small intestine with harmful bacteria leads to earlier and more intense triggering of the symptoms by FODMAPs after food intake, since additional intestinal gases can arise earlier in the digestion process, namely already in the small intestine. In fact, there is convincing evidence that an altered bacterial colonization of the small intestine occurs more frequently in IBS patients than in the unaffected population. However, a direct relationship between the altered intestinal microbiota in these patients and the development of symptoms by increased FODMAP intake with food has not yet been conclusively established.

What happens with FODMAPs in the large bowel?

In the large intestine (colon), FODMAPs are fermented by the resident bacteria. This process generates intestinal gases and other degradation products. The intestinal gases lead to bloating, flatulence and abdominal pain. There are short-chain and long-chain FODMAPs. Short-chain FODMAPs are fermented much more quickly by the intestinal bacteria than the long-chain ones, meaning that fermentation of lactose, for instance, leads to the generation of intestinal gases much faster than fermentation of long-chain FODMAPs.

In addition, fermentation of FODMAPs in the colon produces degradation products which bind water in the intestine and actively cause the intestine to release water into the intestine. Both mechanism lead to loose stools, including diarrhea.

Fermentation in the colon, and the resulting degradation products, cause additional issues such as partial alteration of the intestinal bacterial flora, changes in the colorectal mucosa cells and the inflamm-

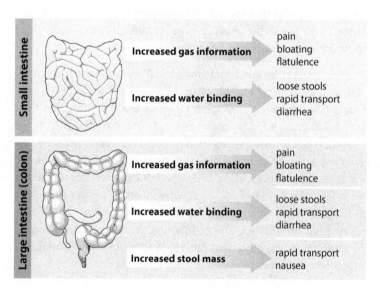

Mechanisms of symptom generation by FODMAPs

atory processes in the colonic wall, resulting in increased permeability of the wall of the colon. This increased permeability, in turn, promotes inflammatory processes of the colorectal wall.

Can the FODMAP effects be demonstrated in humans?

A diet high in FODMAPs leads to an increase in intestinal gasses and hence an increase in flatulence and digestive problems. A scientific study has shown this to hold true for the patients with irritable bowel syndrome as well as for the unaffected persons. It is interesting to note that the amount of intestinal gas produced by a high-FODMAP diet is the same in both healthy people and patients with irritable bowel syndrome, but the patients report more severe symptoms and a more pronounced flatulence. This phenomenon is explained by the hypersensitive gut. Also interesting is the fact that the intestinal flora in people who consume a diet high in FODMAPs is more strongly altered in IBS patients than in the unaffected people. The significance of these changes in the intestinal microbiota is still unclear.

What end-products are produced during fermentation of FODMAPs?

Fermentation of FODMAPs produces gases, short-chain fatty acids and lactic acid. The resulting gases are mainly hydrogen (H_2) and carbon dioxide (CO_2). Ammonia (NH_3), oxygen (O_2), methane (CH_4) and nitrogen (N_2) as well as the foul-smelling gases methanethiol (CH_4S), hydrogen sulfide (H_2S) and dimethyl sulfide ($(CH_3)_2S$) are also produced in slightly smaller quantities. The short-chain fatty acids include acetate, butyrate and propionate, which in some cases also lead to an odor problem.

Are there extra-intestinal FODMAP effects?

Most of the known effects by FODMAPs arise directly in the colon due to fermentation and its end-products. These end-products cause changes directly in the colon, which in turn lead to symptoms. There are, however, indications that individual FODMAPs also cause other effects in our body, at sites distant from the colon.

In patients with irritable bowel syndrome and fructose malabsorption or lactose intolerance, it was observed that a concurrent mild depression was significantly improved by a fructose or lactose-free diet. It remains unclear, however, whether this depression is caused by fructose malabsorption or lactose intolerance, that is to say that it is directly connected with the disease, or whether it is caused by long-term symptoms, over the years, i.e. appearing secondary to the underlying disease.

Significantly better established is the link between the uptake of fructo-oligosaccharides belonging to FODMAPs and the development of heartburn. Fructo-oligosaccharides can aggravate the reflux of the gastric contents and gastric acid into the esophagus, thereby causing heartburn.

How do intestinal gases cause discomfort?

Fermentation of FODMAPs produces gases in large quantities. These gases cause symptoms such as bloating, flatulence and abdominal pain. The precise mechanism of how these gases cause intestinal symptoms is well-established. Various studies have shown that gasses that had been delivered into the intestinal lumen triggered flatulence and abdominal pain.

The severity of the measurable symptoms depends on the amount of intestinal gas. The more intestinal gas and fluid are found in the small and large intestine, the more the intestine is expanded and inflated from the inside, which in turn clinically manifests itself in bloating, flatulence, abdominal pain and loose stools. The frequency of bowel movements is also increased with increased intestinal contents: on the one hand because more stool volume is produced, and on the other hand because the increased intestinal filling stimulates intestinal activity, resulting in a more frequent urge to defecate and actual defecation. The only currently unresolved aspect is how come an excess of FODMAPs leads to constipation and firm stools in a small sub-group of people. Irrespective of a lack of explanation for it, however, patients with firm stools and constipation also benefit from a low-FODMAP diet.

Besides abdominal pain, many patients also report a bloating sensation, and in some bloating is indeed objectively recognized by an increase in abdominal circumference. This effect of intestinal gases on the development of symptoms is not detectable solely in patients with IBS, i.e. those with already existing problems, but also in persons without IBS. The only thing that sets them apart is the stimulus threshold, which makes a certain amount of intestinal gas perceived (sometimes painful).

This mechanism of intestinal gases triggering symptoms is particularly clearly established for intestinal gas in the colon and the distal third of the small intestine. However, gasses are not the only thing that causes an expansion of the intestine from the inside; distension caused by solid or liquid components in the intestinal lumen may also cause symptoms.

This is of high relevance for FODMAPs since bacterial fermentation of the FODMAPs leads to the formation of other bacterial degradation products in addition to gases. These bacterial degradation products cause fluid to flow into the intestinal tract, thereby increasing the liquid and solid intestinal contents. Both contribute to an increased filling of the intestine in addition to the filling by intestinal gases, and intensifies the symptoms. In summary, FODMAPs lead to symptoms or worsening of symptoms through various degradation products.

Without a doubt, our intestine is designed for the absorption of gases, fluids and food components from it into the body. However, if our diet is too high in FODMAPs, intestinal gases are produced too quickly and in too large a quantity. In turn, too much water is bound in the intestine, in particular due to the short-chain FODMAPs and their degradation products. Since our bodies can no longer compensate for this, the unpleasant symptoms arise. The data from scientific studies are unequivocal and speak for the FODMAP diet. Fewer FODMAPs cause less intestinal gases and less intestinal contents, in turn causing fewer digestive problems.

Visceral hypersensitivity

Visceral hypersensitivity, also termed the sensitive gut, is highly pre-valent in all functional bowel disorders, including irritable bowel syn-drome. However, tests for this are not offered in daily clinical practice because the derived information would not contribute to any thera-peutic decisions, meaning that the patients would not benefit from such tests. Sometimes these hypersensitivity tests are carried out in scientific studies. The testing principle is very simple.

A balloon is first inserted into the rectum and gradually inflated. The filling level at which the patient perceives the balloon is called the per-ception threshold. When the balloon is further inflated, the patient starts to feel pain, which is called the pain threshold. These thresholds are measurable in every patient, and they tend to be shifted in patients with irritable bowel syndrome. They perceive the balloon sooner and also the distension is perceived as painful sooner. This is a very un-complicated test that simply and graphically describes what leads to abdominal pain and other symptoms in patients with irritable bowel syndrome.

Patients with irritable bowel syndrome have a more sensitive intestinal tract, rendering them more perceptive to pain.

The origin of the hypersensitivity of the intestine has not been clarified. In the case of irritable bowel syndrome, a variety of causes are considered possible, including hereditary factors, environmental influences and, last but not least, the intestinal flora. Unfortunately, there is as yet no adequate answer to the question as to why visceral hypersensitivity occurs. But the test principle helps us understand another issue. The test balloon is nothing but a substitute for intes-tinal gases. It is the intestinal gas filling that leads to paresthesia and pain in patients with a sensitive bowel or IBS. This explains why the same amount of intestinal gas does not cause any discomfort in a healthy person.

Activity of intestinal muscles and transport velocity

Another point is important in the development of symptoms due to FODMAPs. It is very well known that in patients with IBS, the intestinal wall muscles respond to distension stimuli with increased muscle activity, that is to say, stronger muscle contractions. This leads to abdominal cramps and an increased urge to defecate. For this reason, increased intestinal gases as they occur after FODMAP consumption cause abdominal cramping and frequent bowel movements.

Changes in the intestinal flora

Several clinical studies have shown that the composition of the intestinal flora in patients with irritable bowel syndrome is significantly altered in comparison with the flora of an unaffected person. However, we do not yet know enough about the „normal" composition of the intestinal flora; hence, the changes in the intestinal flora in patients with IBS cannot be classified. For the same reason, it is also not clear what bacteria are associated with what changes, which bacteria are involved in the development of the symptoms, and the consequences of the detected changes in the intestinal flora in patients with irritable bowel syndrome. However, it is conceivable that some bacteria ferment FODMAPs more potently than others; the only thing missing is the evidence that this is so in patients with irritable bowel syndrome, too.

 Patients with IBS display an altered intestinal flora as compared with the healthy people. Hence, it is conceivable that cerain bacteria handle FODMAPs better than others.

It is interesting that the composition of our intestinal flora changes depending on whether we eat a high or low-FODMAP diet. A low-FODMAP diet leads to a reduced presence of various bacteria from the group of *Clostridia*. Some groups of *Clostridia* species are very pathogenic and spoil or poison food; hence, it is conceivable that the changes in the intestinal flora of persons on a low-FODMAP diet contribute to the improvement of the digestive problems.

Are the FODMAP effects detectable?

Yes, for each and every step in the FODMAP hypothesis, there is evidence reflected in human studies. It has been shown that FODMAPs are actually poorly (or not at all) absorbed from the small intestine into the body's circulation and directly enter the colon, where they are fermented by resident bacteria. It has also been demonstrated that this fermentation leads to an increase in the stool volume, in particular by an increase of the liquid components, and that abundant intestinal gas is formed. For individual FODMAPs such as fructose, sorbitol, lactose and fructo-oligosaccharides it has been demonstrated that they can cause symptoms in healthy individuals when they are present in high quantities, while in patients with IBS even in much smaller quantities. Numerous clinical studies have also revealed that the effects of the individual FODMAPs are synergistically augmented when ingested together, as is customary in our mixed diet.

Lactulose, the synthetic FODMAP

Lactulose is an artificial double-sugar consisting of fructose and galactose. In the intestine, lactulose cannot be split into the individual sugars; hence, lactulose cannot be absorbed in the intestine. There are no natural sources of lactulose. Strictly speaking, lactulose is a synthetically produced FODMAP.

The actual use of lactulose is rather interesting. It is used as a laxative and characterized in particular by a very good water-binding capacity in the intestine. Thus, lactulose has a laxative effect and causes the stool to soften. Like the other FODMAPs, lactulose also leads to the formation of intestinal gases by fermentation in the colon. For this reason, flatulence is often reported as a side effect when lactulose is taken, in addition to the mentioned laxative effect and looser stools.

In essence, the effects of the laxative lactulose are the best proof of the FODMAP theory.

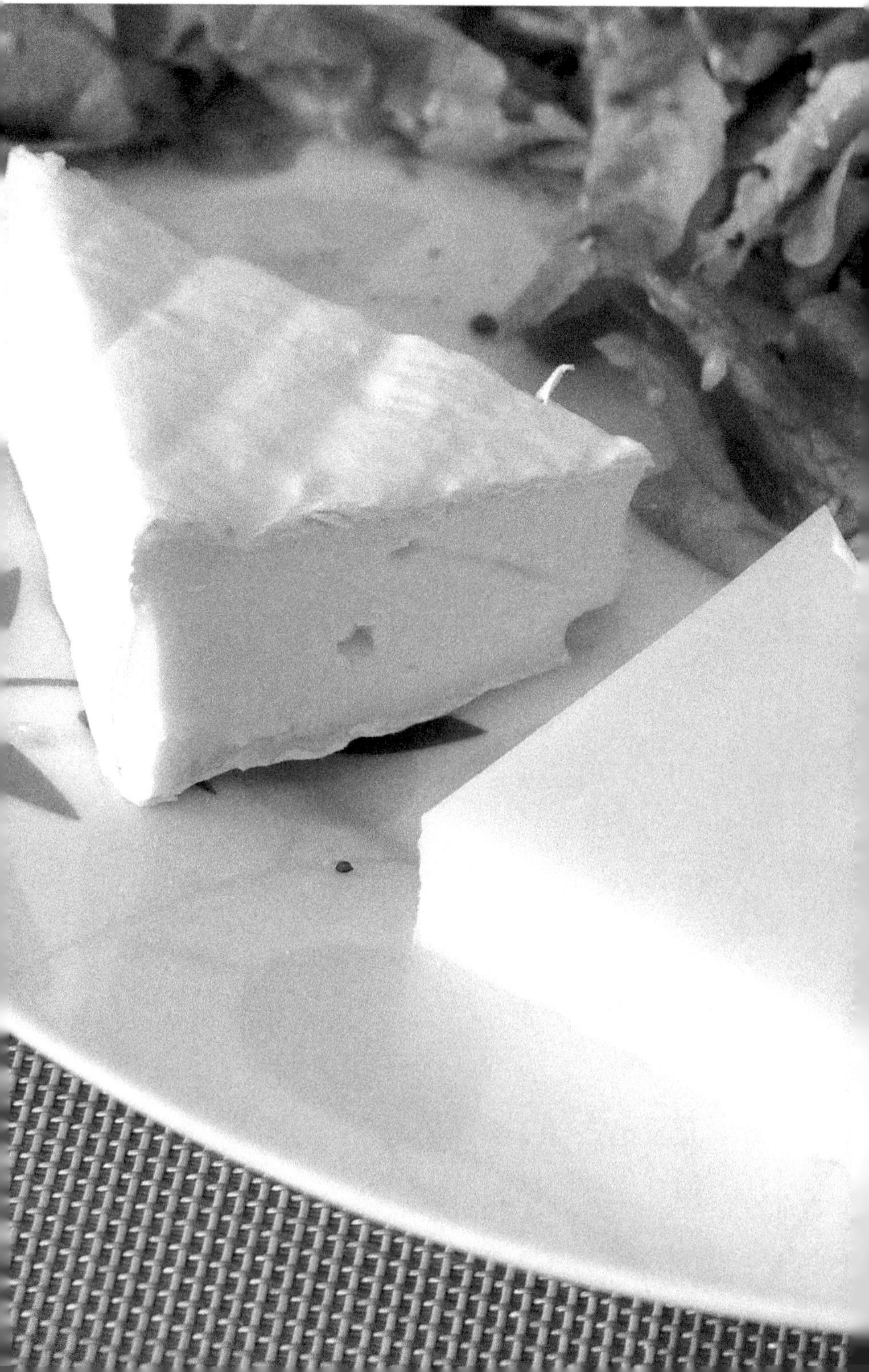

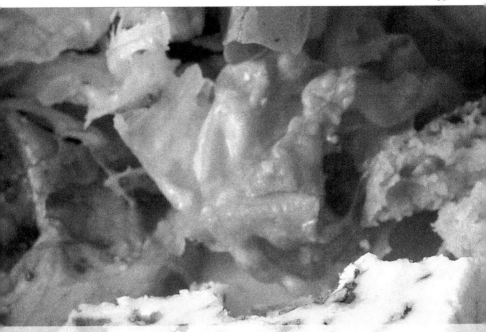

Chapter 3
Who benefits from a low-FODMAP diet?

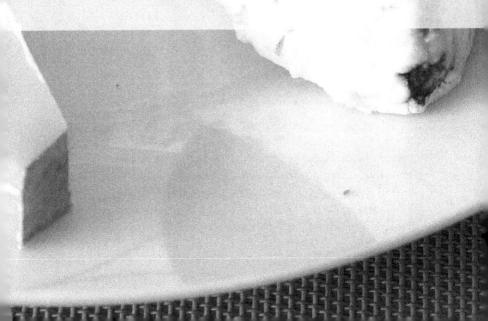

The FODMAP concept is very new and has not yet been studied in many diseases. The low-FODMAP diet has been thoroughly studied in patients with irritable bowel syndrome, and in those with bloating and diarrhea. Patients with other diseases benefit too, but the current study quality is not yet as good. The text below describes the illnesses and symptoms in which a low-FODMAP diet is promising according to our present knowledge.

For whom is a low-FODMAP diet suitable?

FODMAP-diet - definitely beneficial - investigated in clinical studies	FODMAP-diet - beneficial - not yet investigated in clinical studies
Irritable bowel syndrome in children and adults	FODMAP intolerance
Inflammatory bowel disease such as Crohn's disease and ulcerative colitis with symptoms despite well- controlled intestinal inflammation	Non-specific gastrointestinal symptoms (boating, abdominal pain, diarrhea)
Wheat sensitivity (wheat intolerance)	Fructose malabsorption with an inadequate response to a fructose-free diet
Patients who suffer from diarrhea or other symptoms in the hospital	Lactose intolerance with an inadequate response to a lactose-free diet
	Patients in whom colon has been removed and who often have loose or watery stools

Which diseases cause digestive complaints?

A variety of diseases are associated with digestive problems and gastrointestinal symptoms. This Guide is not a substitute for seeing a doctor, and it is important to consult a doctor first in order to prevent serious illness. Often, however, no explanatory causes are found for digestive complaints, and the diagnosis of irritable bowel syndrome is made. In these cases, a low-FODMAP diet is promising. Whether a low-FODMAP diet is promising in cases of digestive problems caused by a diverticular disease of the colon has not yet been established in studies, but when flatulence and loose stools are the chief complaint, it is definitely well worth a try.

Irritable bowel syndrome

Irritable bowel syndrome is a common disease. The patients report bloating, flatulence, abdominal pain and changes in bowel movements. The stool can be too loose, sometimes even watery, or too firm, and defecation may be too frequent or infrequent. These symptoms and changes in bowel movements do not always occur, but rather they can occur only on individual days. It is also not uncommon for the symptoms to appear intermittently or alternately.

The causes of irritable bowel syndrome are not fully understood. In addition to a hereditary component, gastrointestinal infections, environmental factors and nutritional factors also play a role. The interplay of all these factors leads to a markedly inconsistent disease pattern. For this reason, the affected persons often do not know for years what is wrong with them. As a result, they see different specialists and subject themselves to a variety of examinations, sometimes for several years, before the right diagnosis is made.

The diagnosis of irritable bowel syndrome is made when the above-mentioned digestive complaints occur regularly and limit the quality of life. The physician orders examinations to rule out other diseases, which could explain the symptoms. Depending on the main symptom, different forms of progression are distinguished.

They include IBS with diarrhea, IBS with constipation, IBS with abdominal pain, IBS with bloating, and IBS with alternating symptoms. It is important to note that despite the designation according to the main symptom, other digestive symptoms can occur simultaneously.

Various forms of irritable bowel syndrome depending on clinical course:

► IBS with diarrhea
► IBS with constipation
► IBS with abdominal pain
► IBS with bloating
► IBS with alternating symptoms

Treatment of irritable bowel syndrome can be achieved by a variety of measures. In addition to drugs, alternative medicine measures and the low-FODMAP diet are also promising.

Fructose malabsorption and symptoms despite a diet low in fructose

As mentioned earlier in this Guide, fructose malabsorption is an independent disease that can be conclusively diagnosed with a breath test. The treatment includes a diet low in fructose, while a low-FODMAP diet is not necessary in this disease entity. However, some patients with fructose intolerance continue to show signs of indigestion despite a diet low in fructose.

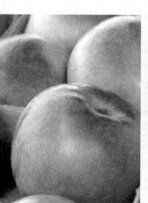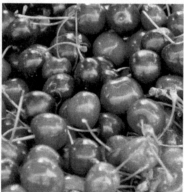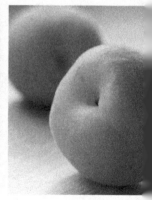

Fructose malabsorption and irritable bowel syndrome may occur simultaneously as well.

This may be due to the fact that fructose malabsorption and IBS are simultaneously present, which occurs more often than one would imagine. Both diseases are common and can therefore occur concurrently. In such a case, it is worthwhile to add a low-FODMAP diet to the low-fructose diet. That said, however, such an „trial" should not be performed for longer than 6–8 weeks, and a continuation of the FODMAP diet is recommended only if you feel that your symptoms are improving significantly.

Lactose intolerance and symptoms despite a diet low in lactose

Lactose intolerance is diagnosed with special breath tests, as described above for fructose malabsorption. Once lactose intolerance has been conclusively diagnosed, the therapy consists of a lactose-free or a lactose-reduced diet. In most patients this leads to a good control of symptoms. In some cases, however, digestive problems persist despite the lactose-free diet. In such a situation, the low-FODMAP diet can be tried. The FODMAP diet should first be maintained for 6–8 weeks. If the symptoms improve, it can be continued. If not, the diet should be discontinued.

Celiac disease

Celiac disease is an autoimmune disease characterized by an immune reaction against gluten, leading to inflammation of the small intestine and subsequently to symptoms such as bloating and diarrhea. In short, when a patient presents with bloating and diarrhea, celiac disease should be considered.

Gluten is a protein found in wheat, rye and barley. Celiac disease is treated with a gluten-free diet. This gluten-free diet, however, clearly differs from the low-FODMAP diet. It is not necessary to eat gluten-free in the context of a low-FODMAP diet, and a strictly gluten-free diet is not recommended unless celiac disease has been unequivocally diagnosed.

Celiac disease is distinguished from wheat allergy and wheat sensitivity using tissue studies of the small intestine and blood tests detecting antibodies against gluten (tissue transglutaminase antibodies). These antibodies prove the existence of celiac disease. Since celiac disease is not directed against wheat, but rather against gluten, the necessary diet is a gluten-free diet, i.e. wheat, rye, and barley-free.

If you have celiac disease, the low-FODMAP diet is not suitable for you. If, however, you still experience digestive problems despite a strictly gluten-free diet, and your doctor cannot find any other cause that explains your symptoms, you may find it helpful to try a low-FODMAP diet as well.

Wheat allergy and wheat sensitivity

There are two disease presentations that are very similar to celiac disease, namely wheat allergy and wheat sensitivity, also called wheat intolerance, which are often confused. The accurate medical term for wheat sensitivity is actually „non-celiac-non-wheat allergy wheat sensitivity". These diseases are confused very frequently since they are characterized by very similar symptoms, they are accompanied by very similar intolerances, namely the intolerance to wheat, and they are treated with very similar measures, namely wheat-free diets. Nevertheless, they are different diseases.

Celiac disease can be distinguished very well from wheat allergy and wheat sensitivity. Wheat allergy is also characterized by the formation of antibodies in the body. However, these antibodies are not directed against gluten, but rather against other wheat proteins such as gliadins and thioredoxins. This disease is a real allergy. However, not all of these antibodies can be detected in clinical laboratory tests, usually only antibodies against gliadin are determined.

In addition to the digestive problems such as bloating, abdominal cramps, abdominal pain, nausea and diarrhea, wheat allergy may additionally present with allergic symptoms of the skin, lungs, eyes and mouth. The diagnosis of wheat allergy is sometimes complex because the serum antibodies we know may be absent. Further diagnostic studies, such as gastroscopy, ileoscopy and colonoscopy may contribute a variety of non-specific clues, but they cannot provide a definitive diagnosis. If you have wheat allergy, the low-FODMAP diet is not a suitable diet for you.

Wheat sensitivity is a disease in which no antibodies are formed and thus no detection with blood tests is possible. The symptoms of wheat sensitivity is more akin to celiac disease. The chief complaint are digestive problems. To make the diagnosis, it is necessary to first exclude celiac disease and wheat allergy.

A carefully kept nutritional symptom diary can lead to the right track. On the other hand, many additional complaints are reported in wheat sensitivity. Muscle, bone and joint problems as well as headache, fatigue, lassitude and concentration problems have been described. Whether all these symptoms actually belong to wheat sensitivity or whether they are part of a more complex, hitherto not fully understood, disease pattern is currently a subject of heated debate.

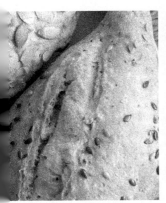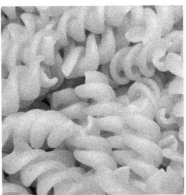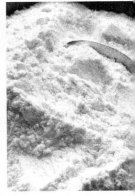

Wheat allergy, wheat sensitivity, and celiac disease are frequently confused due to the similar symptoms, but they are actually three separate diseases.

It is not clarified which components of wheat lead to wheat sensitivity, that is, to hypersensitivity. The trigger is presumably not gluten; hence, the term gluten sensitivity, which was used occasionally in the past, is no longer used. The wheat protein amylase trypsin inhibitor (ATI) is currently strongly suspected of triggering hypersensitivity. The interesting thing about this protein is that it is less present in older wheat varieties than in modern high-performance wheat, i.e. wheat bred with modern methods to bring as high yields as possible. This could be an explanation as to why increasing number of people suffer from wheat sensitivity.

There is a body of evidence in the literature that FODMAPs can trigger symptoms of wheat sensitivity. Very relevant here is a clinical study involving patients with wheat sensitivity, who were treated with a low-FODMAP diet for two weeks. Interestingly, a low-FODMAP diet reduced the symptoms in all patients. The second part of the study is

Differences between celiac disease, wheat allergy, and wheat sensitivity

	Celiac disease	Wheat allergy	Wheat sensitivity
Period from food intake to symptoms	Weeks to years	Hours to days	Hours to days
Blood tests	Transglutaminase antibodies	Wheat IgE antibodies (with limitations)	Gliadin-Antibodies
Skin test	No	Yes	No
Inflammation of the small intestine	marked	mild (possible)	Unclear, possibly mild
Long-term sequelae	possible	unknown	unknown
Incidence	1:100	1:100 assumed	1:50 – 1:100 assumed
Diet	gluten-free	wheat-free	low-FODMAP or low-wheat

highly interesting as well: After two weeks of the low-FODMAP diet, one group of patients received a bit of gluten added to their diet, while the other group received a lot of gluten. In both groups, symptoms appeared in some patients, but it did not matter whether they received little or much gluten. This implies that gluten is not responsible for the symptoms of wheat sensitivity.

Currently, there are still significant gaps in our understanding of wheat sensitivity. Further research is needed. Some experts even question the existence of this disease. According to the results of the clinical trials, however, instituting a low-FODMAP diet is worth a try in cases of confirmed or suspected wheat sensitivity. A gluten-free diet does not seem to benefit patients with wheat sensitivity, and there is no adequate information on whether a strictly wheat-free diet is effective.

Inflammatory bowel diseases: Crohn's disease and ulcerative colitis

Inflammatory bowel diseases such as Crohn's disease and ulcerative colitis are characterized by inflammation of the small intestine. In severe cases, they are treated with drugs. In some patients with inflammatory bowel diseases, however, digestive problems persist, although the inflammation of the gut responds well to drug treatment which curtails the intestinal inflammation and normalizes inflammatory parameters in the blood. This is then a case of functional intestinal complaints associated with an inflammatory bowel disease.

Such functional intestinal complaints are 2 to 3 times as frequent in patients with a well-treated inflammatory bowel disease as in the normal population. If no other causes are found, it is assumed that these functional complaints correspond to those of irritable bowel syndrome, prompting the same treatment. Therefore, in this case, instituting a low-FODMAP diet is well worth a try.

Intestinal surgery

For various medical reasons, it may be necessary to partially or completely remove the colon. As a result of this, digestive discomfort with bloating, abdominal pain, flatulence and loose stools often occur. A low-FODMAP diet is helpful in this case in order to get these symptoms under control or at the very least to achieve a significant relief.

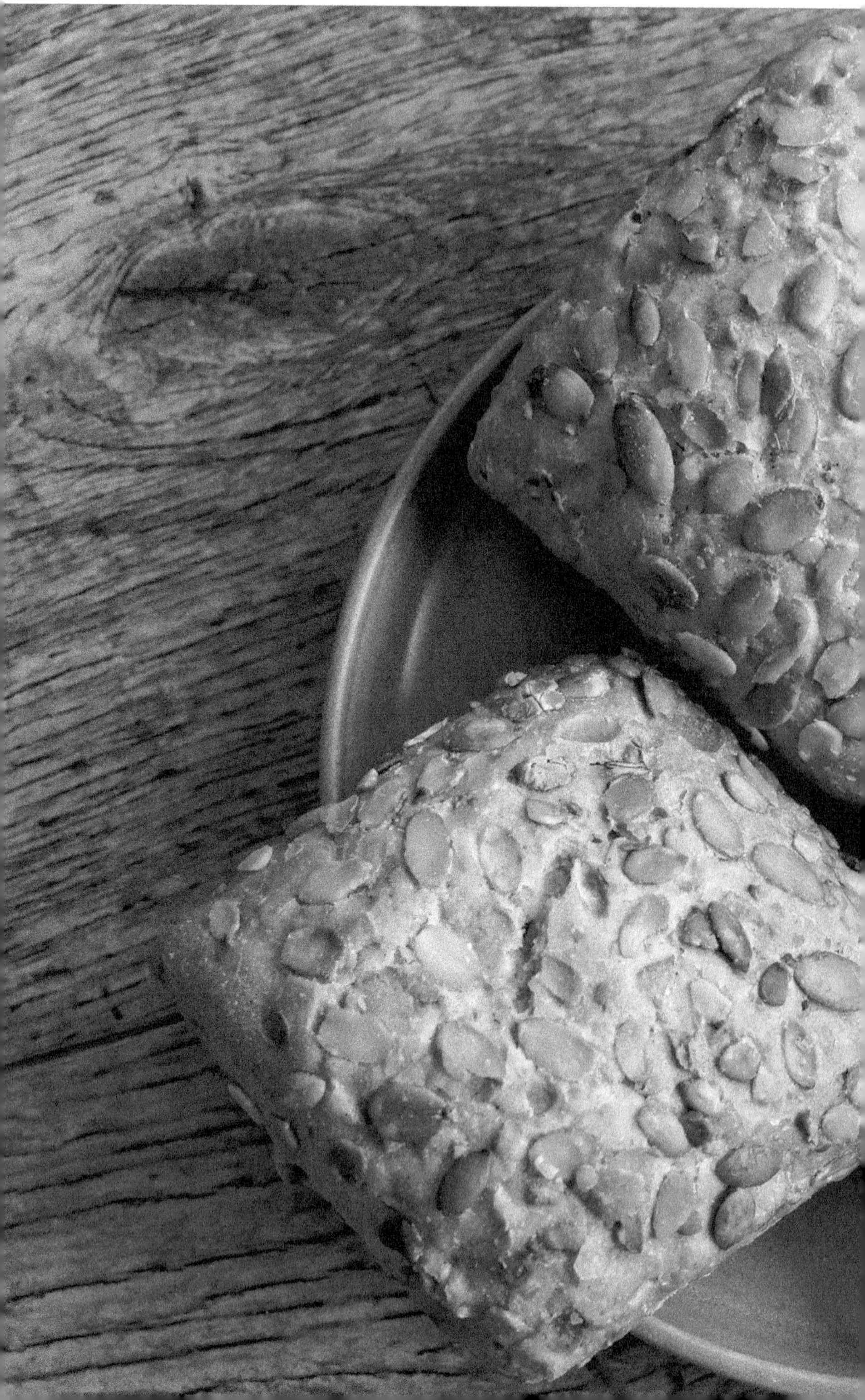

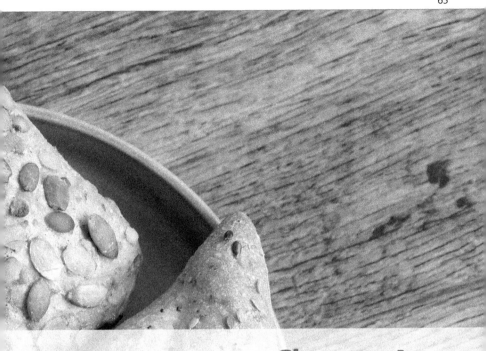

Chapter 4
Understanding the
FODMAP diet

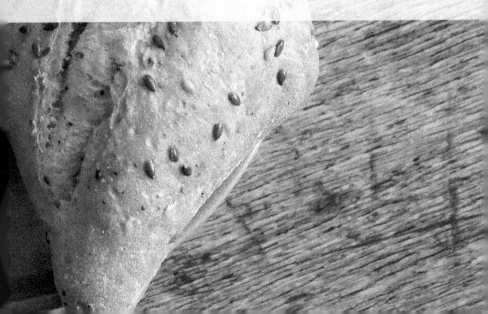

Many patients with digestive problems such as bloating, flatulence, abdominal pain, loose stools or even diarrhea are convinced that the diet is the culprit for their symptoms, or that certain food ingredients are the direct cause of their symptoms. The affected persons observe that the symptoms occur shortly after food intake or that the symptoms occur repeatedly after the intake of certain foods.

Patients often report that after getting up, and during the first hours of the day (in connection with breakfast), they experience increased bowel movements and more frequent loose to watery stools. During the course of the day, bowel movements normalize. The next morning, however, everything starts all over again. However, such observation often has nothing to do with the composition of food. Rather, the culprit are increased gastrointestinal reflexes in a sensitive gut because the activity of the digestive system is usually highest in the morning hours and immediately after a meal, while it decreases during the day and between meals.

Another common observation is that the symptoms occur directly after eating certain foods. This may indicate an intolerance. But here too it should be noted that symptoms that occur directly after food intake are not caused by an intolerance. Foods that actually cause an intolerance must first pass through the stomach in order to enter the small intestine. Only there do such intolerances lead to symptoms. In essence, it takes a certain time before symptoms appear.

Unraveling intolerances

For these reasons, detecting food intolerances is sometimes a complex task. In the case of a severe intolerance with serious and promptly manifest symptoms, it is somewhat easier to recognize the correlation and to initiate the necessary diagnostic work-up. On the other hand, a mild intolerance with mild symptoms often makes it very difficult to recognize the correlation and to commence the required work-up.

In order to be absolutely certain that a person suffers from a food intolerance, it is helpful to have the patient keep a nutritional symptom diary in order to get a better overall picture. In such a diary, all meals,

Nutritional symptom diary

Date:

Time	Food and drinks consumed	Symptoms	Other comments
(Please document for each event)	(please document the amount, preparation form and any herbs)	(please be as specific as possible, indicating the duration and severity of the symptom(s), on a scale from 1 to 10 (10 = none, 10= very severe)	(e.g. medications, vitamins, stress)

Template of a nutritional symptom diarys

the individual food ingredients, and the exact time of food intake are recorded over a limited period of time, typically four weeks; in addition, it is documented whether the person experienced symptoms or not, and if so which complaints occurred at what time.

If a food intolerance is unequivocally established, a corresponding diet should be followed.

Diets for irritable bowel syndrome

If a patient has irritable bowel syndrome, and food allergy or intolerance has been excluded, the decision as to whether a particular diet should be followed or not, and which one, is not quite so simple. Since irritable bowel syndrome is a disease with many causes and triggers, there has been no standardized diet beneficial to all patients.

The medical literature contains a variety of dietary approaches designed to alleviate the symptoms of irritable bowel syndrome or individual symptoms affecting the bowel. Numerous diets are based on the fact that a diet designed to help with food intolerances may also be used to improve symptoms such as bloating or changes in bowel movements in patients with IBS. Although many of these diets follow very clear and rational explanatory models, it is difficult to prove that these dietary changes actually lead to symptom relief.

These concepts work in individual cases or in small patient groups. This is why they are occasionally recommended. However, most of these recommendations were not tested in large patient groups. Therefore, no standardized IBS diet has been proposed thus far. This has now fundamentally changed with the advent of a low-FODMAP diet.

The gradual path to a low-FODMAP diet

If a dietary therapy is to be carried out in symptomatic patients, it is advisable to proceed in three steps. This step-by-step approach is delineated in great detail by the British National Institute for Health and Care Excellence (NICE Institute).

This is a three-step process. If the first step is not helpful, proceed to the second step. However, if the symptoms improve, there is no need to proceed to the next step.

1st step: General nutritional recommendations

2nd step: Low-FODMAP diet

3rd step: Elimination diet

We start with some general nutritional recommendations. The recommendations can be found on the next page.

It may be a good idea to keep a nutritional symptom diary for a period of four weeks in order to recognize individual food sensitivities and to adjust the dietary plan accordingly. These general recommendations are typically implemented for eight weeks. If an adequate symptom relief is attained, the diet can be continued. However, If these general measures are not sufficient, the next step is to start a diet which omits poorly digestible foods. This is where the low-FODMAP diet comes into play, because the low-FODMAP diet has been most thoroughly clinically tried and tested for IBS. Hence, it is recommended in this case. According to the results of clinical trials, the low-FODMAP diet will benefit all patients with irritable bowel syndrome, regardless of whether they pass stools that are too loose or too solid. Clinical studies offer concrete evidence for the improvement of bloating, flatulence and abdominal pain.

Most patients report an improvement in stool consistency while on a low-FODMAP diet. Patients with diarrhea have fewer bowel movements and can expect to pass firmer stools. A treatment trial with a low-FODMAP diet should be performed for 6–8 weeks, like any other dietary trial.

Resorting to the third recommendation, which is a strict elimination diet, is justified only in a few isolated cases that fail to respond to a low-FODMAP diet. However, the elimination diet should not be carried out without consulting a doctor or nutritionist, and is therefore beyond the scope of this Guide.

Nutritional recommendations for the symptomatic treatment of bloating, abdominal pain and loose stools

▶ Eat your meals regularly, typically three main meals and, if necessary, one to two (light) snacks.

▶ Take enough time to eat your food in a peaceful environment, avoid eating in a rush, or eating while walking or standing.

▶ Drink sufficient amounts of fluid, at least 1.5 liters distributed throughout the day, ideally water or tea, and avoid caffeinated drinks.

▶ Limit the consumption of coffee and black tea to a maximum of 3 cups a day.

▶ Avoid alcoholic or carbonated drinks.

▶ Limit the consumption of fresh fruit to a maximum of three servings per day (each with a maximum of 100 g).

▶ Eat more oats and linseed (1 teaspoon / day) if you suffer from bloating and flatulence.

▶ Avoid artificial sweeteners if you have diarrhea or loose stools; these are often contained in beverages and low-calorie foods.

▶ Avoid resistant and retrograded starch (see page 74).

What makes the FODMAP diet credible?

There are numerous nutritional recommendations that promise relief from bloating, abdominal pain and altered bowel movements. Why should I believe that the low-FODMAP diet is any better? There are several reasons for it.

Initially, a concept was developed for the low-FODMAP diet based on the question of what pathological changes in the bowel cause symptoms. The next step involved identifying those food ingredients that cause changes such as increased intestinal gas, increased abdominal pain or watery stools. All these food ingredients have been summarized under the umbrella term „FODMAPs".

Subsequently, the low-FODMAP diet was tested in clinical trials to see whether the symptoms indeed improve. These trials are up-to-date and of high quality. The patients with symptoms were randomized (i.e. assigned randomly) into two groups: one group received a standard Western diet, and the other group a low-FODMAP diet. Patients did not know which diet they were receiving. Such studies enable a dietary concept to be tested without bias. The FODMAP diet has demonstrated its superiority in these studies, and has since been recommended by specialist associations.

 The low-FODMAP diet is based on a scientific concept that was tested and confirmed in various clinical studies.

Are FODMAPs unhealthy or even dangerous?

The clear-cut answer to this question is „No". FODMAPs are neither unhealthy nor dangerous. FODMAPs are naturally-occurring food ingredients; in some cases they are even added to industrially processed foods. FODMAPs become an issue only when they are ingested in excessive amounts. Our gastrointestinal tract can deal with them to a certain extent. Since FODMAPs are for the most part very poorly digestible, they are not absorbed in the small intestine and enter the colon, where they are digested by the resident bacteria. FODMAPs are literally „fast food" for our gut bacteria.

As a rule, FODMAPs are no problem for our bodies – as long as everything works well. Only if too many FODMAPs arrive in the colon, the resident bacteria have too many FODMAPs to digest. Consequently, too many bacterial digestive products overwhelm our intestines. These include intestinal gases. For people with a more robust physique, this turns out to be no problem, the body can handle it. For those with a more sensitive gut, however, the increased intestinal gases are already a problem, and they readily develop symptoms. In this way, an essentially healthy person can turn into a patient with frequent digestive complaints if his/her diet contains too many FODMAPs. Likewise, a patient with well-controlled digestive symptoms can turn into a patient with uncontrollable, recalcitrant symptoms.

What happens when a healthy person follows a low-FODMAP diet?

Nothing. Since healthy people have no complaints, they cannot improve. The diet is tested on healthy subjects, and a healthy person perceives the changes in the type of food consumed, but that is it.

Is there a risk of nutritional deficiencies?

No. On the one hand, the low-FODMAP diet only reduces and does not completely eliminate FODMAPs; on the other hand, FODMAPs are not essential food ingredients, which means that a deficiency is expected neither in the healthy nor in patients with symptoms, even if the FODMAP share in their diet is reduced to the very minimum.

How many meals a day should I eat?

When on a low-FODMAP diet, you should eat as normally as possible. This also applies to the number of meals eaten. The general nutritional recommendations stipulate three main meals and, if necessary, one or two (light) snacks, ideally consisting of small quantities of fruit. These guidelines should be followed when on a low-FODMAP diet as well. If this is not enough for you, please refer to the FODMAP table to identify foods low in FODMAPs that can serve as additional snacks.

Is the positive effect of the low-FODMAP diet proven?

There are numerous dietary and nutritional suggestions for improving symptoms of irritable bowel syndrome or digestive symptoms of other causes. Some of these recommendations are well-supported by clinical trials, others less well. However, most of the diets are based on traditions or expert opinions and have not been studied in clinical trials, at least not in well-designed trials. This does not mean that all these diets are ineffective, but only that their efficacy is not adequately documented.

The situation regarding evidence is somewhat different for the low-FODMAP diet. This dietary concept was initially proposed by an Australian expert panel as a hypothesis. The hypothesis was essentially based on a variety of nutritional symptom analyses published by various authors and newly interpreted by the said group of experts. Next, this low-FODMAP dietary concept was tested on small patient groups. As it had turned out that the concept works and that a low-FODMAP diet actually offers symptom relief, elaborate clinical trials were initiated involving a large number of patients with irritable bowel syndrome. To date, six clinical trials furnished data on the low-FODMAP diet.

In the largest study, the patients received either a low-FODMAP diet or a normal diet for three weeks. The patients were again randomized (i.e. randomly assigned) to a dietary plan. After three weeks of therapy, the patients on one diet received the other diet for three weeks afterwards. During the entire study period, symptoms such as abdominal pain, abdominal cramps, bloating and diarrhea were recorded. The remarkable thing about this large clinical study was that neither the patients nor their study doctors knew whether the patients were in the low-FODMAP or the normal diet group at any point in time. In medicine, such studies are called double-blind studies because no one knows – neither the doctor nor the patient – which therapy a particular patient is receiving. It is precisely this design that makes double-blind studies so meaningful, since the study results cannot be influenced consciously or unconsciously in such a study.

To date (year 2016), the concept of a low-FODMAP diet has been studied in countless studies in many countries around the world. In doing so, the FODMAP diet was adapted to the local diet and, in particular, locally different serving sizes. Thus, the concept can be examined in studies in very different countries.

Resistant starch, retrograded starch: What are they?

Resistant starch is starch that cannot be digested by the digestive enzymes in the small intestine, and therefore enters the colon where it can cause symptoms after conversion by the resident bacteria.

High quantities of resistant strength are found, for example, in green bananas and in certain corn varieties.

Retrograded starch is starch that becomes indigestible by heating and subsequent cooling. Retrograded starch is found particularly after heating foods rich in starch such as potatoes and cereal products, as well as in industrially processed foods. We do not yet know the content of resistant starch in most foods. The generation of resistant starch is very variable and depends on the food, on the type of preparation, duration and temperature, as well as on many other circumstances.

What you should know about fiber

A frequent recommendation in the past was that the amount of dietary fiber should be increased in patients with irritable bowel syndrome. However, this recommendation does not work for all affected persons since many dietary fibers arrive in the colon in an undigested form, and are decomposed by resident bacteria. This applies in particular to the water-insoluble plant fiber which we take in with fruits, vegetables, cereals and bran. During bacterial decomposition, intestinal gases are generated, and these intestinal gases cause symptoms. Therefore, dietary fiber, especially the water-insoluble dietary fiber, often leads to a paradoxical, counterproductive effect in patients with digestive complaints by making their symptoms stronger rather than weaker.

> Water-soluble fiber, such as psyllium and linseed, bind water in the intestine and thus act as stool-regulating agents, their effects best unfolded in the granulated, crushed or ground form.

The current state-of-the-art recommendation is that the diet should be supplemented with water-soluble dietary fibers in patients with symptoms of irritable bowel syndrome. In the intestine, the water-soluble dietary fibers bind abundant water and lead to better stool consistency, regular bowel movements, and thus symptom relief. Water-soluble fibers are less potently decomposed by bacteria in the colon, thereby generating less additional intestinal gas. Therefore, water-soluble dietary fibers such as psyllium or psyllium husks are considered stool-regulating products.

Psyllium products which are available in pharmacies and health food stores in various forms are produced from the Indian plantain. Psyllium husks can bind up to 50 times their weight of water in the intestine. The effect of granulated or ground psyllium is better than the effect of untreated one. In addition to psyllium, oat is also rich in water-soluble fiber and is suitable for fiber fortification and additional water binding. Linseed is also rich in water-soluble fiber, but should only be crushed or best ground, since it is otherwise ineffective and appears undigested in the stool.

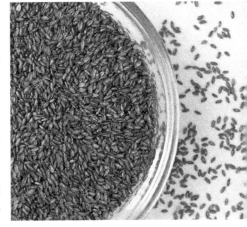

The influence of the composition of the intestinal flora on the digestion of dietary fiber is not clear. What we know, however, is that patients with digestive problems

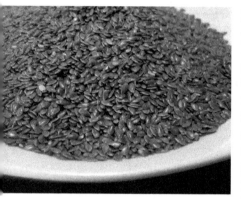

produce more intestinal gases from dietary fiber, report increased flatulence, have more severe abdominal pain, and a different composition of the intestinal flora than patients without digestive problems. Although it is still too early to name the bacteria responsible for increased intestinal gas production, bacteria with fun names like Bacillus uniformis, Bilophila wadsworthia and Parabacteroides distasonis are among the suspects.

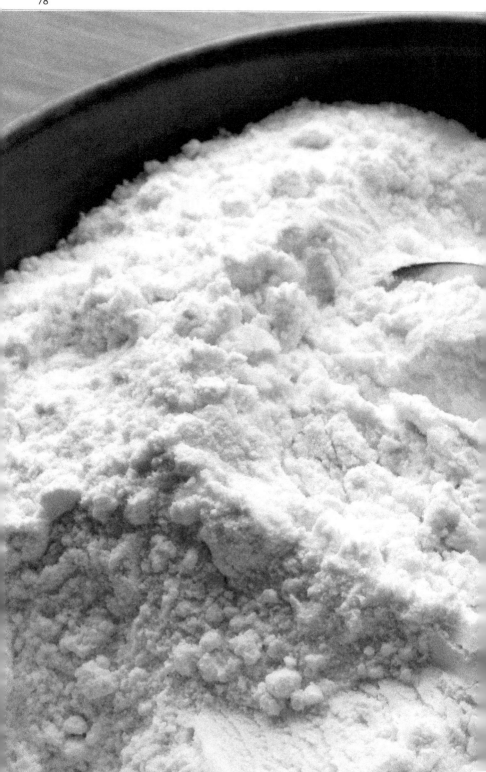

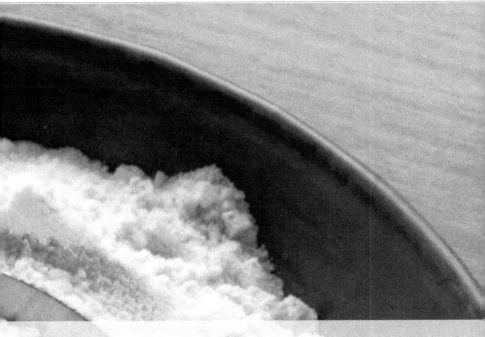

Chapter 5
The first step is always the hardest

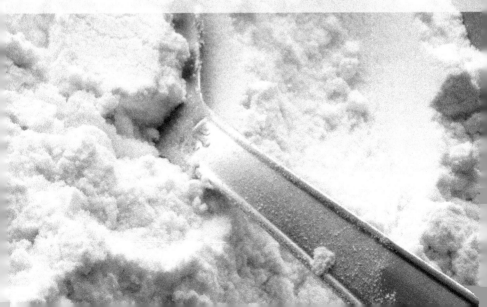

In the previous chapters, you learned about the basics of the low-FODMAP diet. Now let's implement this knowledge. It is nearly impossible to obtain information on each food in detail, and to measure the content of the individual FODMAPs in these foods. This is not necessary either. As the name implies, the low-FODMAP diet is not about eating no FODMAPs at all because this is not possible, but rather, it is about identifying foods low in FODMAPs and avoiding foods that are high in FODMAPs.

Since various FODMAPs are contained in different quantities in different foodstuffs, it is the the overall assessment of the individual foodstuffs that counts. The content of various FODMAPs is included in this overall assessment; subsequently, the food is classified as low or high in FODMAPs. A lemon, for example, which contains moderate amounts of fructose and traces of polyols, is classified as low in FODMAPs overall, since it contains only a low share from the other FODMAP groups. The following table shows the assessment of FODMAP content of individual foods.

In order to be able to create a successful low-FODMAP diet for yourself, please refer to the tables of the next double-page listing foods high in FODMAPs and foods low in FODMAPs. These must be either selected or avoided.

FODMAP content of individual foods, and how the overall assessment is arrived at

	Fructose	Lactose	Oligo-saccharides	Polyols	Overall assessment
Rice	traces	traces	none	none	low in FODMAPs
Pear	much	none	none	much	high in FODMAPs
Lemon	moderate	none	traces	traces	low in FODMAPs
Cherries	much	none	traces	traces	high in FODMAPs
Strawberries	moderate	none	traces	moderate	low in FODMAPs

To simplify your grocery shopping, we have reprinted these tables in the cover of this book for you to copy and take along.

Please note that the tables are only an aid providing a rough guidance on food assessment.

The size of the servings also plays a role in tolerability since you take in more FODMAPs with a larger serving.

For example, you may be able to eat a very small amount of a food high in FODMAPs without experiencing symptoms, but you will experience discomfort when eating a very large quantity of a food that is actually classified as low in FODMAPs.

How can I reduce FODMAPs in my diet?

The FODMAP content depends on where you live, your culture and the local characteristics of your diet. Our Western lifestyle is characterized by a diet that is particularly rich in fructose, fructans and polyols.

Initially, the foods high in FODMAPs should be avoided, but later they can be consumed again in small quantities. On the other hand, you can mix and match foods low in FODMAPs at will to create your diet.

If you have decided to try the low-FODMAP diet, strongly consider doing grocery shopping yourself, preparing your own meals, and preparing them from as few different foods as possible. This will simplify your low-FODMAP diet.

Foods that contain lots of FODMAPs and whose consumption should be reduced

Fruits	Vegetables and legumes	Cereals and grain products	Dairy products and milk substitutes	Other foods
Banana (ripe)	Artichoke	Bread, cereals, pastries, semolina, flakes, pasta, flour etc. from:	Butter milk	**Sweeteners**
Apple	Asparagus		Coffee cream	Corn sirup
Apricot	Beans (except green beans)		Condensed milk	Fructose sirup
Avocado	Beetroot	• amaranth	Ice milk	Honey
Blackberries	Black salsifiy	• barley	Cream	Maple sirup
Cherries	Cauliflower	• rye	Creamer	Sugar substitutes (-it und -ol)
Currant	Garlic	• triticale	Creme cheese	
Figs	Girasole	• unripe spelt grain	Heavy sour cream	**Chocolate**
Grapefruit	Green onion (white part)	• wheat	Kefir	Carob chocolate
Guave, unripe	Leek (white part)		Milk powder	Milk chocolate
Kaki (persimmons)	Lentils *	Lupin flour	Quark	White chocolate
Lychees	Mushrooms		Sour cream	**Nuts**
Mango	Onion	Bulgur	Soy milk * (from soybeans)	Cashew nuts
Mirabelle	Peas	Couscous	Tsatsiki	Pistachios
Nashi-pear Nectarine	Savoy	Wheat germ	Whey	**Alcohol, drinks**
Peach	Shallot		Whey powder	Beer (more than one glass)
Pear	Soybeans		Yogurt	Liqueur
Plums	Sweet corn		**Cheese**	Port Wine
Pomegranate	Sweet peas		Farmer cheese	Rum
Sugar banana, ripe	Sweet potato		Halloumi	Sherry
Watermelon			Mascarpone	Wine, sparkling wine (semi-dry; sweet)
Canned fruits			Whey cheese	
Cocoa water Dried fruits				**Vegetable protein**
Fruit juices				Silken tofu

* FODMAP content varies, depending on the processing

Foods that contain few FODMAPs and are suitable for a low-FODMAP diet

Fruits	Vegetables and legumes	Cereals and grain products	Dairy products and milk substitutes	Other foods
Banana (firm)	Alpha alpha	Bread, cereals, pastries, semolina, flakes, pasta, flour, etc. made from:	Butter	**Sweetener**
Blueberries	Broccoli (ss)		Coconut milk	
Cantaloupe	Brussel sprout (ss)		Lactose-free milk	Aspartam
Cantaloupe melon	Carrot		Lactose-free dairy products	Maple sirup
Carambola	Celeriac (ss)			Stevia
Chestnuts	Celery (ss)	• buckwheat	Oleo (margarine)	Sugar sirup
Clementine	Chard	• corn (polenta)	Soy milk * (from soy protein)	Sugar (white, brown)
Coconut (ss)	Chickpeas * (ss)	• millet		**Chocolate**
Durian	Chicorée salad	• oats*		Dark chocolate
Galia melon	Chillies	• quinoa	**Cheese**	
Grapes	Chinese cabbage	• rice	Brie	**Nuts and seeds**
Guave, ripe	Chives	• spelt flour *	Camembert	always fewer than 15 pieces of:
Kiwi	Corn * (ss)	• tapioca	Cheddar	• almonds
Kumquat	Cucumber		Chester	• brazil nuts
Lemon	Eggplant	Potato starch	Edamer	• hazelnuts
Lime	Fennel		Emmentaler	• macadamia
Maracuja	Ginger	Corn chips (ss)	Feta	• pecan
Muskmelon	Green beans	Cornflakes	Gorgonzola	• walnuts
Orange	Green onion (green part)	Popcorn	Gouda	always less than 15 g of:
Papaya	Hokkaido	Potato chips (ss)	Hard cheese	• chia seeds
Pineapple	Kohlrabi		Harzer cheese	• peanuts
Pineapple-melon	Leek		Mild, full-flat cheese	• pumpkin seeds
Pitaya	Maniok (ss)		Mountain cheese	• sesame seeds
Prickly pear	Okra		Mozzarella	• sunflower seeds
Raspberries	Olives		Parmesan	**Alcohol, drinks**
Rhubarb	Parsnip		Pecorino	Beer (not more than 1 glass)
Starfruit	Pepper		Raclette	Wine (dry)
Strawberries	Potato		Ricotta	**Meat and plant protein**
Sweet chestnuts	Radish		Tilsiter	Eggs, fish and meat
Tangerine	Radishes			Seafood
	Red cabbage			Tofu (solid, without additions)
	Salad/lettuce			
	Soybean sprouts	(ss) = small serving		**Öle und Soßen**
	Spaghetti squash	* FODMAP content varies depending on the processing		Vinegar
	Spinach			Vegetable oils
	Tomato			Mustard
	White cabbage			Soy sauce
	Zucchini			

Indigestion
no further treatment necessary
(seeing a doctor is an option)

Preparation
Decision to adopt the low-FODMAP-diet
± nutritional counseling

Phase 1 – Strict diet
6 – 8 weeks of a strict low-FODMAP-diet

Phase 2 – Re-introduction
Determine the FODMAP tolerance threshold
for individual foodstuffs (preferably)
or
re-introduce individual FODMAP groups (second choice)

Phase 3 – Long-term dietary approach
Individual FODMAP diet, consuming a low FODMAP content
and knowing your tolerance threshold for individual foods

Strategic approach to the low-FODMAP diet

Ready-made meals, ready-to-serve sauces and the like are best avoided because their FODMAP content is difficult to control. Since it is not possible to know the FODMAP content especially of fresh fruits and vegetables, it is a good idea to take along a copy of the FODMAP lists when grocery shopping in order to be able to distinguish foods that are low in FODMAPs from those that are high in FODMAPs.

Low-FODMAP diet, phase 1: Strictly low in FODMAPs

The first phase of the low-FODMAP diet lasts 6 to 8 weeks. At this time, you should strictly adhere to your low-FODMAP diet in order to obtain maximum therapeutic success. Choose only foods low in FODMAPs from the food tables, and prepare your own meals. As you can see from the tables, there are plenty of foods available, you need not worry about having to eat a monotonous diet.

> The FODMAP diet is not a very restrictive one. Even in the strict phase 1, nutritional deficiencies are not expected.

To make phase 1 of the FODMAP diet as easy on yourself as possible, see page 86 for a replacement table. At this stage, you should select only foods listed in the green table and strictly avoid those in the red table. In the second part of this book, you will find some recipes that will help you get started with your low-FODMAP diet. You will find recipe suggestions for the main meals – breakfast, lunch and dinner. You will also find suggestions for starters and desserts. Since the topic of bread requires a lot of attention, you will also find recipes for making your own bread and for the bread baking machine.

> The strict phase 1 of the low-FODMAP diet is not a life-long diet.

In the first 6–8 weeks, it is about getting rid of the digestive problems and getting to know the maximum possible success. During this phase you will also develop greater awareness of food and ways to prepare it. This more conscious approach often adds to a more positive attitude towards life. When you have successfully mastered this period, you will proceed to Diet Phase 2.

> The strict Phase 1 lasts only 6 to 8 weeks . You can look forward to a more liberal Phase 2.

Replacement table: High-FODMAP foods are replaced by low-FODMAP ones (selection)

Food group	Foods high in FODMAPs ...	replaced by alternatives low in FODMAPs
Fruit	Apple, apricot, avocado, banana (ripe), blackberries, cherries, currants, grapefruit, lychees, mango, nashi pear, nectarine, peach, pear, persimmon, plums, watermelon	Banana (firm), blueberries, clementine, grapes, honeymelon, kiwi, lime, lemon, maracuja, orange, papaya, pineapple melon, raspberries rhubarb, strawberries, tangerine
Vegetables and legumes	Artichoke, asparagus, beans, beetroot, cabbage, cauliflower, (all except green string beans), garlic, green onion (white part), leek (white part), lentils, mushrooms, peas, savoy cabbage soybeans, sugar peas, sweetcorn, sweet potato	Alfalfa, beans, broccoli (small serving), Brussel sprouts (small serving), carrot, celery (small serving), chard, chickpeas (small serving, soak and pour off water), chicory lettuce, chinese cabbage, chives, cucumber, eggplant, fennel, ginger, green onion (green part), green string, Hokkaido kohlrabi, leeks (green part), lettuce, okra, olives, parsnips, peppers, potato, pumpkin, radish, soy sprouts, spinach, tomato, white cabbage, zucchini
Flour, grains	Amaranth, barley, lupine, rye, triticale, wheat products (wheat semolina, wheat germ, wheat bran, bulgur, couscous)	Products made of buckwheat, corn, millet oats, potato flour, quinoa, rice, tapioca (FODMAP content may vary depending on processing)
Dairy products	Condensed milk, cream, cream cheese, ice cream, mascarpone, milk, milk powder, sour cream, yogurt	Lactose-free milk, lactose-free dairy products, Brie, Camembert, Cheddar, Feta, hard cheese, mozzarella, Parmesan
Sweetening agents	Agave sirup, corn sirup, fructose sirup, honey, sugar substitutes ending in -it or ol (mannitol, sorbitol, maltitol, xylitol)	Aspartame, maple sirup, rice sirup, sugar (white, brown), sugar sirup, stevia
Nuts and seeds	Cashew nuts, pistachios	all other nuts and seeds in small quantities

FODMAP Diet Phase 2 – Re-introduction of foods

In the first few weeks, you learned how your digestive problems improve if you follow an optimal low-FODMAP diet. However, the long-term goal is not to permanently adhere to a strict low-FODMAP diet. Phase 2 of the diet is about re-introducing a wider variety of possible foods to make your diet richer and more diverse. This can be accomplished in a variety of ways.

Design your own FODMAP diet.

The more care you take in Phase 2 when re-introducing different food groups/foods, the more you will benefit from your low-FODMAP diet in the long run.

Reintroducing individual foods

One way is to slowly re-introduce individual foods into the diet and gradually increase the amount of these foods. These steps should proceed slowly, each step ideally takes 3–4 days, since the intestine is a rather inert organ and it can take 3–4 days from food intake to the emergence of symptoms. This will tell you the maximum amount of a foodstuff high in FODMAPs that you still tolerate well enough without developing digestive symptoms.

It is of utmost importance to investigate each foodstuff separately. For any food that is high in FODMAPs, and which you cannot do without, you can learn what amount your body will tolerate without digestive discomfort. These tolerability thresholds are very different. Your goal should be to figure out your personal threshold. If you find that some foods cause digestive problems in very small amounts already, you should remove them from your diet for good.

Reintroducing FODMAP categories

It is up to you to decide whether you want to start reintroducing individual foods or different FODMAP categories. The introduction of individual foodstuffs is easier, so this procedure is recommended.

If you want to test your tolerability of FODMAP groups, the following foods are suitable for a tolerance test for the various FODMAP groups.

This testing is best accomplished if you have a written plan to follow.

Be sure to test only individual foods or FODMAP groups, otherwise you may loose track and can no longer correctly assign symptoms or complaints.

Fructose tolerance is tested using two spoonfuls of honey, which is very high in fructose, or alternatively, three apples. A glass of whole milk is suitable for testing lactose tolerance. To test your fructane tolerance, use an onion or one or two cloves of garlic. Galactan tolerance is tested with a lentil dish. Testing polyol tolerability is somewhat more difficult, since polyols and fructose occur together in most natural products. A test with five pieces of sorbitol and mannitol-containing chewing gum appears suitable.

FODMAP Diet Phase 3 – The long-term dietary approach

Once Phase 2 is completed, you begin your personal diet. You know those foods high in FODMAPs that you can tolerate and also those that you cannot tolerate. You know your tolerance threshold for individual high-FODMAP foods. You will find that you hardly tolerate some high-FODMAP foods even in very small quantities. Some patients realize at the end of Phase 2 that they can enjoy an almost normal diet and that they cannot tolerate only isolated high-FODMAP foods. Others, on the other hand, realize that they do not tolerate polyols at all, but that they are more or less OK with all other FODMAPs. The goal is to find your individual, diverse and balanced diet, that enables you to stay permanently symptom-free.

In general, you should treat all foods whose FODMAP content you do not know, as well as all industrially processed foods that do not provide sufficient information on the ingredients, as foods high in FOD-MAPs. You will probably be able to evaluate industrially processed mixed foods in the long term, and to gradually reintroduce them into your diet, if this is still something you want to do.

 Hands off food whose FODMAP content you do not know and cannot assess!!

You will most likely slide back into a high-FODMAP diet when you create your individual diet. This is not uncommon, there are ups and downs in our lives. Simply re-examine your diet to identify dietary errors, and adjust it.

If the low-FODMAP diet does not help

In some cases, the low-FODMAP diet brings no improvement or only a partial improvement of the digestive problems. There are various reasons for this. One possible reason is that an individual high-FOD-MAP foodstuff slipped into your diet. In order to get to the bottom of this, again carefully review the FODMAP food list to identify any such dietary errors and adjust the diet accordingly.

Another reason why the low-FODMAP diet does not help may be that another disorder or intolerance is responsible for your digestive problems, such as intolerance to food additives such as gluten or other naturally occurring food chemicals such as amygdalin in fruit cores, glycoalkaloids such as solanine in potatoes, lectins in beans, cucurbitacins in zucchini and oxalic acid in rhubarb leaves. Intolerances to these substances are, however, rare.

What about cheese?

Individual cheese varieties contain FODMAPs in different quantities. The essential FODMAP in cheese is lactose. Lactose contained in milk is decomposed during cheese production by the enzyme lactase, which is mostly derived from bacteria during the production of cheese. Therefore, the FODMAP/lactose content in cheese varieties with a long aging time is lower than in cheese varieties with a little to no aging time.

Cheese varieties with a long aging time such as hard cheese, feta cheese, Camembert and Brie, are well-suited for a low-FODMAP diet. Cheese varieties with a short aging time such as cream cheese and cottage cheese are high in FODMAPs because of their high lactose content, and therefore not very suitable.

You should know the lactose content of the different types of cheese in order to assess their FODMAP content. Refer to the following table for the lactose content of different types of cheese. In the upper half of the table you can find the most suitable cheese varieties (low in lactose), while in the lower half of the table you will find unsuitable types of cheese (high in lactose). Since the lactose content in various products can fluctuate, the values in the table are only a rough guide.

What about other dairy products?

It is important to know the lactose content of other dairy products as well. Different dairy products contain lactose in different amounts. In the upper part of the table you will find dairy products with a low lactose content, and in the lower part products with a high lactose content. Since the lactose content in the various products can fluctuate, the values in this table are also merely a rough guide.

What other foods contain lactose?

Lactose is found in many industrially processed foods because lactose has a positive effect on the consistency of the food. It is a favorable filler and it becomes brownish in color when heated. This brownish color is a reason why lactose is added in the production of sausages. Particularly in the case of industrially processed foods, it is important to study the ingredients. Small quantities of lactose are also consumed with medicines since lactose is used as a carrier and filler in drug manufacturing. The lactose content of some drugs is indeed very high, but since tablets are absorbed only in small quantities little lactose is absorbed in this way.

Lactose content in cheese in g/100 g

Low lactose content	
Brie	0,1–0,2
Group of cheeses produced in the Alps	< 0,1
Camembert	0,1–0,2
Chester	< 0,1
Edamer	< 0,1
Emmentaler	< 0,1
Feta	0,5
Gouda	< 0,1
Harzer cheese	< 0,1
Mild, full-fat cheese	< 0,1–1
Mozzarella	< 0,1
Parmesan	< 0,1
Raclette	< 0,1
Ricotta	0,3
Tilsiter	< 0,1
High lactose content	
Cream cheese	2–4
Cottage cheese	3,3

Lactose content in dairy products in g/100 g

Low lactose content	
Butter	0,6
High lactose content	
Buttermilk	4
Condensed milk	9,3
Cow milk	4,5–5,5
Cream	3–4
Goat milk	4,2
Ice cream	5–7
Kefir	3,5–6
Milk powder	35–50
Quark	2–4
Sour cream	2–3
Yogurt	3–3,5

What you should know about yogurt?

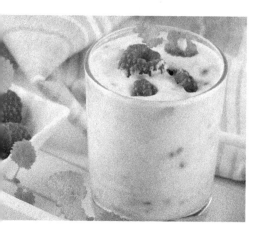

Yogurt is high in lactose. However, if you do not want to do eliminate yogurt, you can look out for a few things that make some yogurts better tolerated than others. The FODMAP in yogurt is lactose, and its content can vary considerably in yogurt. The fluctuations depend on the manufacturing conditions. Lactose is degraded by the enzyme lactase in yogurt bacteria cultures. The longer these cultures can work, the lower the lactose content of the final product. Using your own yogurt machine, you can influence the time of production and let the yogurt cultures work 14 hours, or even as long as 18 hours, instead of 10 hours.

This makes yogurt lower in lactose and therefore more digestible. When purchasing yogurt, make sure that it has not been pasteurized or heated, because this kills off all bacteria. Buy yogurt that contains living bacteria since they continue to split lactose in your intestines and thus exert a positive effect on digestion.

If you choose to make your own yoghurt, you can use lactose-free milk. In this milk, the lactose is split into glucose and galactose. These two sugars do not cause digestive problems. Because of the glucose and galactose content, this yogurt tastes somewhat sweeter. It is important to note that for the production of yogurt made from lactose-free milk, a different yogurt culture is needed than for yogurt made from cow's milk. This yogurt culture is available at food health stores; alternatively, you can start your yogurt culture with cultures made from fresh, non-heat treated, lactose-free yogurt.

Is the FODMAP share in our diet increasing?

Yes, the share of FODMAPs in our diet is increasing for a variety of reasons. On the one hand, our dietary habits are changing towards more industrially processed foods and soft drinks. Both are sources of additional fructose. Fructose is used for sweetening here. But our consumption of fruits and fruit juices is also changing. Eating more fruit goes hand in hand with higher a consumption of FODMAPs, and FODMAPs in fruit juices are absorbed in very high concentrations.

The changes in consumption are particularly evident in the case of various sugars. While the consumption of table sugar is declining and the consumption of lactose remains stable, the consumption of fructose is steadily increasing. Likewise, the increase in the consumption of polyols, i.e. sugar substitutes, in our diet can be explained by our altered nutritional behavior. The rising consumption of beverages, especially sweet drinks, and the rising consumption of low-calorie foodstuffs, are driving a higher consumption of sugar substitutes. This is especially evident in the case of beverages. 25 years ago, we did not know low-calorie or calorie-free drinks, meanwhile they have become standard.

Another reason for the increase in FODMAPs in our diet is the trend towards industrially processed foods and fast food. These products are high in FODMAPs due to their high content of fructose and polyols.

The share of FODMAPs in our diet is increasing due to:

► more industrially processed foods
► more soft drinks
► more low-calorie foods
► more snacks high in FODMAPs

Another trend in our diet leads to an increase in the daily FODMAP intake. A large part of the daily energy intake is nowadays provided by snacks, sweets or power bars. All these „intermediate meals" are high in FODMAPs. The type of foods we tend to consume on a daily basis has also changed. The share of pasta products, pizzas, cakes, cereals, pastries and products with a high fruit content has more than doubled over the last 20 years.

The amount of fructans consumed has also changed. Fructans are undoubtedly beneficial in food production. They improve the texture and stability of the food. Occasionally, food is marketed as a beneficial product due to its fructan content and hence fiber content. The fructan-potato is an example. In the end, however, all these fructan additions also change the daily consumed FODMAP quantity. While most cereal products contain a high share of fructans, the rice plant cannot synthesize fructans. Rice is therefore fructan-free. This is one reason why rice diets are very well tolerated by patients with digestive problems.

Foods with added fructans can be identified, for example, by the label oligosaccharides, fructo-oligosaccharides or chicory.

What about meat, fish, chicken, fats and oils?

Sources of protein such as meat, fish and chicken, as well as fats and oils, contain hardly any FODMAPs. This is because these foods contain hardly any carbohydrates. Therefore, these foods can be freely

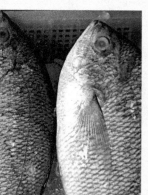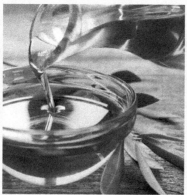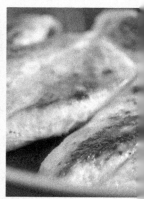

Fish, fats and oils, and meat are low in FODMAPs or FODMAP-free.
Sauces, marinades and dough coat, however, may contain FODMAPs

consumed by patients on a low-FODMAP diet. It should, however, be noted that the ingredients added during processing such as sauces, marinades or a dough coat do contain FODMAPs. Hence, their FODMAP content should be considered.

How to assess the ready-made products?

You will encounter difficulties in assessing the FODMAP content of the ready-to-use or ready-made products. Finished products which are offered in cans, dried or also frozen, but also sauces and dressings, contain a lot of FODMAPs and what is more, they often contain retrograded starch. Currently, the FODMAP content of these dishes is not indicated on the packaging.

It is best to avoid such products if you are on a low-FODMAP diet, since this will allow you to have the best control over your diet. If you do not want to do without such dishes, you should carefully study the ingredients to assess the food. Please pay particular attention to ingredients such as fructose, sweeteners, onion and garlic, as these are often added in large amounts.

How many FODMAPs are in hot drinks?

Coffee contains only a low amount of FODMAPs and can be consumed as part of the diet. An exception is instant coffee, which is high in FODMAPs. It should be noted, however, that the added coffee cream or the added milk is high in FODMAPs and should be avoided. If you drink your coffee with milk, use lactose-free milk or a low-FODMAP substitute milk instead of cow's milk that is high in FODMAPs.

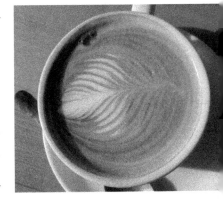

Apart from the FODMAP content assessment, you should also remember that caffeine stimulates peristalsis and can therefore cause or intensify digestive problems. Therefore, the daily amount of coffee should be limited to a maximum of three cups, or even less if you suffer from digestive problems, regardless of the FOD-MAP content. No FODMAP assessment has yet been carried out for coffee substitute products; due to their chicory or malt content, these substitute products are, however, to be regarded as high in FODMAPs.

The evaluation of teas is not as easy as the evaluation of coffee because there are so many varieties. Peppermint tea, green tea, herbal tea and black tea are considered to be low in FODMAPs.

Tea varieties high in FODMAPs are oolong tea, fennel tea and chamomile tea. In addition, the longer the tea bag sits in the cup, the higher the FODMAP content. This is important for chai tea and some herbal teas, so beware of leaving the tea bag in too long.

Cocoa is low in FODMAPs and therefore suitable, if water, rice milk or lactose-free milk is used in the preparation of the hot beverage. When cow's milk is used, it must be taken into account that cow's milk is high in FODMAPs.

How many FODMAPs are in chocolate?

Cocoa is low in FODMAPs and contributes little to the FODMAP content of chocolate. The FODMAPs in chocolate come from lactose. Therefore, dark and bitter chocolates, i.e. chocolates with a high cocoa content, are well-suited, while milk chocolate and white chocolate should best be avoided.

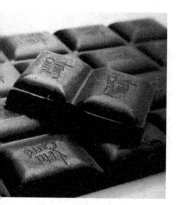

How many FODMAPs are contained in sweets and soft drinks?

Large amounts of sugar substitutes are hiding in sweets. Sugar substitutes of the polyol type are frequently used. Next time you buy a chewing gum or peppermint drops, review the package and you will find polyols listed. A chewing gum probably does not cause any di-

FODMAP content of teas

Low in FODMAPs	Medium in FODMAPs	High in FODMAPs
Black tea (tea bag left in for a short time)	Black tea (tea bag left in for a long time)	Chamomile tea
Chai tea (tea bag left in for a short time)	Chai tea (tea bag left in for a long time)	Fennel tea
Dandelion tea (tea bag left in for a short time)	Dandelion tea (tea bag left in for a long time)	Herbal tea (tea bag left in for a long time)
Green tea		Oolong tea
Herbal tea (tea bag left in for a short time)		
Peppermint tea		
White tea		

gestive problems, but several of these sweets spread throughout the day contribute significantly to the FODMAP burden. The same applies to low-calorie soft drinks. Frequently, polyols are used as sugar substitutes in these drinks.

Does food preparation/processing change the FODMAP content?

The content of FODMAPs in a foodstuff changes with the preparation. Strong heating results in the decomposition of FODMAPs and thus a reduction in the FODMAP content. Factors such as the preparation temperature, the type (cooking, roasting, microwave) and the duration of the preparation all play a role. The extent to which the FODMAP content is changed by the different methods of preparation is unknown for most foodstuffs. Hence, the preparation is currently not yet addressed by the nutritional recommendations. This is likely to change in the future.

It is interesting that canned foods can release part of the FODMAPs, the so-called water-soluble FODMAPs, into the liquid used in the canning process. If vinegar is contained in the preserving liquid, this effect is further intensified by the acid contained therein. If, for example, canned onions are served, the liquid should be poured off in order to remove at least some of the FODMAPs.

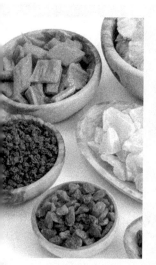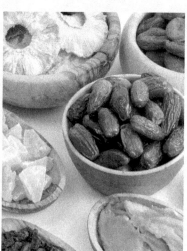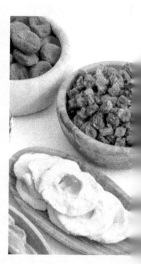

When fruits are dried, the share on FODMAPs per unit of weight increases. Often, additional FODMAPs, such as fructans, are generated by drying.

However, the FODMAP content of certain foods can also increase during preparation, such as when drying fruits. Drying not only deprives the fruit of water, which results in an increase in FODMAPs per unit weight, but it can also result in additional FODMAPs such as fructans, which are not contained in the fresh fruit. For this reason, you should exercise caution especially with dried fruits during the low-FODMAP diet, and be very careful when re-introducing food in phase 2.

How do I replace onions and garlic?

It is not easy to eliminate onions and garlic from our diet. Onions and garlic are needed in many recipes as flavorers or flavor enhancers, and we have gotten used to the good taste. Unfortunately, onions and garlic are very high in FODMAPs and should best be avoided, or consumed in very small amounts when on the diet.

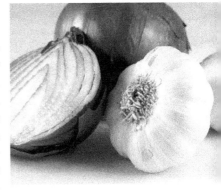

If you do not want to do without onions and garlic, more precisely their fine taste, use a trick. FODMAPs are hardly soluble in oil. You can fry onions and garlic in oil and then remove them from the oil after a short time. The taste is partly transferred to the oil that can be used to prepare dishes, but the high-FODMAP onion and garlic themselves are not consumed. If this is too cumbersome, you can also buy oils that contain onion or garlic flavor. In the case of clear oils, only the taste, but not the onion and garlic, or their FODMAPs, is included. Another way to replace garlic and onion is to use the Ayurvedic spice hing (asafetida) which, unlike onions and garlic, does not leave odors.

What type of bread is low in FODMAPs?

The FODMAP content of bread depends mainly on the flour used. While bread made from wheat, barley or rye flour is considered to be high in FODMAPs and should be avoided, bread made from oatmeal or spelt flour using leaven is relatively low in FODMAPs.

Bread dough that is prepared according to the traditional leavening method, i.e. using yeasts in combination with lactobacilli with a longer leavening time, is somewhat lower in FODMAPs since the yeasts and lactobacilli degrade a larger share of FODMAPs contained in the grain, thereby reducing the FODMAP content. Ask your baker for leavening times and select bread made of flour that is low in FODMAPs and prepared according to the traditional leavening method.

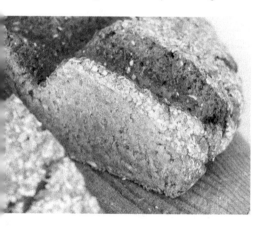

An elegant way to control the FODMAP content of bread is to prepare it yourself. In doing so, you can use grain low in FODMAPs or use alternatives low in FODMAPs such as corn flour, rice flour, or potato starch. In the above table there are numerous alternatives from which bread can be made. If you have nothing against square bread, you can simplify your low-FODMAP life with a bread baking machine. In 2–3 minutes, all the ingredients are mixed together, and the built-in time switches simplify your life and provide you with fresh bread for breakfast that will bolster your quality of life in addition to providing you with a FODMAP-free alternative. Since you do not need to eat entirely FODMAP-free, but merely low in FODMAPs, you need to replace only a part of the wheat flour with, for example, oatmeal. Such breads taste better than, for example, gluten-free breads.

FODMAP content of grain

Low in FODMAPs	High in FODMAPs
Oatmeal	Barley flour
Spelt flour *	Rye flour
* FODMAP content depends on the preparation	Triticale flour
	Unripe spelt grain
	Wheat flour

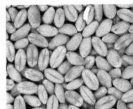

FODMAP content of grain alternatives

Low-FODMAP alternatives	Unsuitable alternative
Arrowroot	Amaranth
Buckwheat	Lupine flour
Corn starch/ corn flour	Pea flour
Millet	
Potato starch/ potato flour	
Quinoa	
Rice flour	
Tapioka starch (from cassava)	

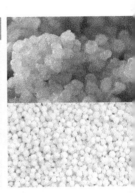

Dietary fiber

Dietary fibers are an important part of the diet. They serve to regulate bowel function and bowel volume. The ability of the dietary fiber to bind water in the intestine plays a role in this process. Dietary fiber is a type of carbohydrate that your body cannot digest; it usually comes from plant sources. More on pages 74 to 76.

Bulking agents, binders and stabilizers

Bulking agents, binders and stabilizers are added to foodstuffs to improve their texture. Most of these substances are not FODMAPs, so you do not need to limit them. This applies particularly to agar agar, carrageenan and gelatin. Pectin, xanthan gum and guar gum (E 412), as well as other stabilizers, cause bloating when consumed in large quantities. Hence, you should limit their consumption to a reasonable level.

Sweeteners

Sweetning is easy in the low-FODMAP diet. You should simply avoid all artificial sweeteners that are polyols. These sweeteners end with the letters -ol, and you will find their alternative names and their

FODMAP content of sweeteners

Low in FODMAPs		High in FODMAPs	
Acesulfame K	E 950	Erythrite (erythritol)	E 968
Aspartame	E 951	Glycerol	E 422
Aspartame-Acesulfame	E 962	Isomalt (Isomaltol)	E 953
Cyclamate	E 952	Lactit (Lactitol)	E 966
Neohesperidin DC	E 959	Maltit (Maltitol)	E 965
Neotame	E 961	Mannit (Mannitol)	E 421
Saccharine	E 954	Sorbit (Sorbitol)	E 420
Stevia	E 960	Xylit (Xylitol)	E 967
Sucralose	E 955		
Thaumatin	E 957		

E-number for food labeling listed in the following table. Other sweeteners such as the natural sweetener Stevia (E 960) and sweeteners not ending in -ol, e.g. aspartame (E 951), may be used.

If you do not use sweeteners but prefer natural sugars, you should use sucrose-based sugars (granulated sugar) or glucose-based sugars (glucose, dextrose). Maple sirup, cane sirup and sugar beet sirup are also suitable. Honey and corn sirup are not suitable for sweetening for they both contain a high fructose content.

Spices and herbs

Spices and herbs are used only in small quantities in the preparation of meals and are therefore not restricted. Many of the spices have also not yet been investigated for their FODMAP content. Ready-to-serve seasonings and sauces should be avoided due to the large number of ingredients that are sometimes poorly identifiable. It is also best to avoid stock cubes, clear soup powders and seasoning sauces such as soy sauce, particularly larger quantities thereof, while smaller amounts are OK. By contrast, you are fee to use anise, basil, cayenne pepper, curry, dill, ginger, cardamom, chervil, coriander, cumin, liquorice, lavender, marjoram, mint, nutmeg, cloves, oregano, peppers, parsley, pepper, thyme, chives, mustard, vanilla, juniper, cinnamon and lemongrass. You can season various dishes with fresh or dried spices and make them even more delicious.

No FODMAP-free life, please! The handling of ready-to-serve products, pastries and drinks

There is no such thing as a FODMAP-free life, and it is not necessary either. The diet should be low in FODMAPs, but not FODMAP-free, which is also not possible. Phase 1 of the diet is strictly low in FODMAPs, while phase 2 is gradually more liberal in terms of restrictions, which means that you will try to re-introduce individual foods high in FODMAPs into your diet.

This is the moment when the question arises as to how to deal with our normal Western diet. The individual foods listed in the tables are very easy to avoid or consume. It is more difficult to permanently avoid industrially processed mixed food. Very few of us really want that. A few simple tips will help you incorporate industrially processed foods, pastries and drinks into your low-FODMAP life.

Sauces and dressings

Sauces and dressings can be found in every refrigerator. It is hard to imagine a barbecue steak without barbecue sauce. You do not have to do without it! Just be sure to take much less dressing, the stress being on „much less". The steak does not have to float in sauce for you to enjoy the taste of it, and a fresh salad with just a touch of dressing simply tastes better.

Take note of the ingredients and avoid FODMAPs that you recognize. Since the exact quantities are usually not declared, you will have to try several products until you find the one that is most acceptable to you, including in terms of quantity. Health food stores regularly offer numerous sauces, dressings and seasonings that are lactose-free and gluten-free. These are suitable for a low-FODMAP diet because at least some of the FODMAPs are removed.

Baking and baked goods

Baking is certainly one of the biggest challenges because it is extremely difficult to find low-FODMAP cereal flour replacement products. This applies to baking cakes and bread, as well as all other foodstuffs where flour is used. There are many substitute flours, and you have learned about them at the beginning of this book. But not a single one of these substitute flours can really replace cereal flour and gluten contained in it. Therefore, different strategies are needed to deal with this situation. One strategy is to avoid such baked goods as much as possible, and later on in phase 2 of the diet find out how much of these baking/flour products you can tolerate.

Ready-made gluten-free flour mixtures

Another strategy is to find substitute flours such as gluten-free flours. This strategy is especially suitable for those who simply adore pastries and flour products. However, always check which flours and which additives are used, as there are also gluten-free substitute flours classified as high in FODMAPs. Some shops offer gluten-free flours at a cheaper price, especially if they are bought in larger quantities. These ready-made substitute flours can be used for baking just like wheat flour. The ready-made substitute flour usually consists of corn flour and rice flour, potato starch, corn starch and an adhesive (guar gum, carob kernel flour or xanthan gum). The ready-made substitute flour is slightly more expensive than wheat flour, but cheaper than the next strategy, which is:

Flour mixtures low in FODMAPs

For breads and pastries

500 g of rice flour

250 g of soy flour *

125 g of potato starch

125 g of corn starch

2 tsp of xanthan gum

For breads and pastries

450 g of rice flourl

50 g of grated hazelnuts

250 g of corn starch

175 g of soy flour *

100 g of tapioca flour

3 tsp of guar gum

For cakes and pastries with egg

450 g of rice flour

50 g of grated hazelnuts

250 g of corn starch

250 g of potato starch

3 tsp of carob gum

* Soy flour contains oligosaccharides. In small quantities, however, most patients with irritable bowel syndrome tolerate it well. Test your individual tolerance threshold.

Making your own substitute flour

The next possible strategy is to mix your substitute flour yourself. You will need a mixture of at least three different flours.

Flour mixtures for bread

For breads or firmer baked products, a possible mixture consists of two parts of rice flour, one part of corn starch, one part of corn flour or soy flour, and two coated teaspoons of substitute gluten per 500 grams of flour. Xanthan, guar gum or carob gum may be used as a substitute gluten. 2 tsp xanthan correspond to approx. 3 tsp guar gum or 3 tsp carob gum. Xanthan gives a rubbery texture, which is not for everyone, while guar gum and carob gum impart a less solid texture. Depending on the firmness, the amounts of these substitute gluten are to be increased or decreased to suit your taste. Corn starch can be found in every supermarket because the starch we usually buy at the supermarket is corn starch. Corn starch can alternatively be replaced by potato starch. Potato starch is called potato flour in many supermarkets.

Flour mixture for cakes and pastries with egg

For cakes with baked eggs, a flour mixture of one part of soy flour, one part of corn starch and two parts of rice flour can also be used.

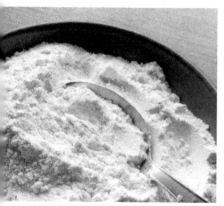

The more different flours you mix, the more similar the characteristics of your flour will resemble those of wheat flour. For example, there are three possible flours on page 105. However, those who find this mixing too cumbersome can obtain gluten-free flours.

For pastries such as Christmas cookies, it is often helpful to increase the share of rice flour a bit. Tastes are different, so you are free to experiment a bit with flour. You will find that baked goods from substitute flour dry out more quickly. If you want your products to be slightly more moist, you can replace a portion of the rice flour with ground hazelnuts.

Drinks

There are non-alcoholic and alcoholic drinks. Drinking only water, ideally mildly carbonated or non-carbonated, would be most compatible with a low-FODMAP diet. Carbonated water is not suitable for your bowels.

Fruit and vegetable juices are high in FODMAPs since they are concentrated. If you drink fruit and vegetable juice, be sure to choose low-FODMAP variants, limit the amount to half a glass and dilute the juice with water, then you'll derive more benefit. In moderation, you do not have to do without orange juice.

If you like to drink milk, it will be hard on you. Try to keep consumption to a minimum or to change to alternatives such as lactose-free milk or rice milk. Admittedly, however, they do not taste the same.

Lemonades, and especially lemonades high in fructose or substitute sugars, are unsuitable. More information can be found in the earlier „Fructose" section of this Guide, as well as in the section „How many FODMAPs are contained in sweets and soft drinks?".

The assessment of warm and hot drinks can be found in the section „How many FODMAPs are in hot beverages?" of this Guide.

As for alcoholic beverages, alcohol should generally be consumed only in moderation or not at all. If you want an alcoholic drink, then beer is rather unsuitable because of the grain and malt content. It should be drunk in small quantities, i.e. a small glass at the most. Wine and sparkling wines are high in FODMAPs, with the FODMAP content rising with the sweetness level. So if you absolutely must have a glass of wine, then select one that is as dry as possible. Other spirits are harmless, but such high-percentage spirits are also not consumed in large quantities. Exercise caution when drinking mixed alcoholic drinks, paying particular attention to the other ingredients.

Is the low-FODMAP diet compatible with other diets??

The low-FODMAP diet is generally compatible with most other diets because you have a wide range of foods to choose from. The situation may become intricate, however, if you have to consume foods high in FODMAPs due to another illness. An example is diabetes because it often requires sugar substitutes that are high in FODMAPs. Another example are liver diseases where special diets are to be observed. If you have to follow a special diet for medical reasons, you should consult a nutritionist before starting the low-FODMAP as part of your individual diet plan.

FODMAPs and the vegetarian or vegan diet

This also applies, with certain limitations, to people who are strictly vegan or vegetarian. A vegan or vegetarian diet is only partially compatible with a low-FODMAP diet, because dairy products and legumes that are high in FODMAPs are frequently consumed in order to meet the protein requirements of vegetarians. Vegetarians and vegans have to plan their diets very carefully. In order to avoid deficiencies, they may have to adopt a less strict low-FODMAP diet. Nutritional counseling is recommended in order to avoid deficiencies.

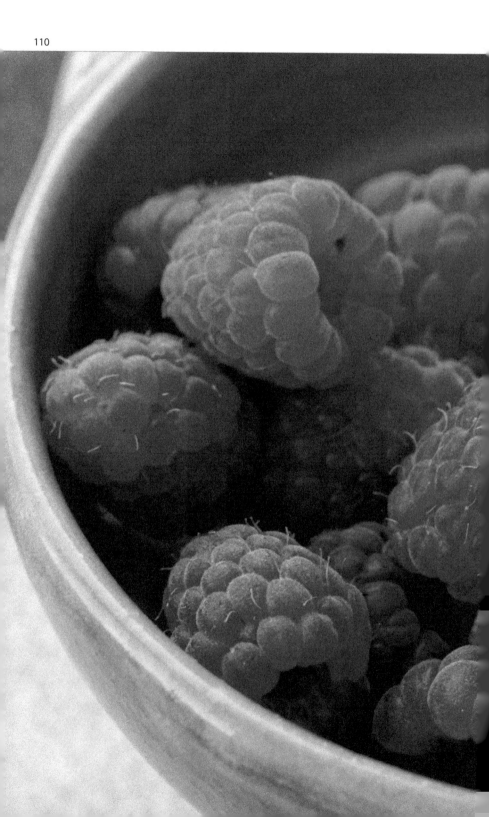

Chapter 6
Recipes

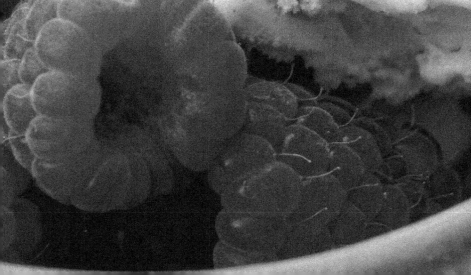

In this chapter you will find some recipe suggestions to get you started. This is not a high-end cookbook, but easy-to-implement suggestions as a stepping stone to a low-FODMAP lifestyle.

Let yourself be inspired by the recipes and take the suggestions as a starting point for your own creations. Everyone's taste is a little different. Therefore, you can and should adjust the recipes to your own taste.

The same applies to individual ingredients. Adapted to what you have in stock, you can exchange ingredients that you do not particularly like with low-FODMAP ingredients and create a novel taste. For example, you can replace oatmeal with buckwheat flakes, and broccoli with Brussels sprouts. Likewise, you can replace maple sirup with sugarcane sirup. The two sirups have a slightly different taste so choose the one that you prefer. If you adapt the recipes to your own taste, make sure that the replacement food is also low in FODMAPs, then you are on the safe side. To replace, for example, oat flakes with wheat flakes would not be such a good idea .

The recipes are meant for 2–3 persons, except for most of desserts which are meant for a party of 4. Since you usually buy 2 bananas in the shop and not 175 grams of bananas, I have provided information on the ingredients as they are usually bought. I personally find this more practical.

Only in the first 6–8 weeks of your low-FODMAP diet (Phase 1) should you select foods that are as low in FODMAPs as possible. Afterwards, in Phase 2 of the low-FODMAP diet, you can re-introduce some foods that are higher in FODMAPs into the diet, and get to know your tolerance thresholds.

Most recipe suggestions are suitable for Phase 1. An exception is the hummus recipe on page 132. In the strictly low-FODMAP phase, you should eat only a small amount of it. In terms of grain and lactose content, you can customize your diet in Phase 2, and depending on how much milk sugar you can tolerate, it may not be necessary to consume only lactose-free products. The same applies to bread and pastries. Most patients will not need to use wheat, barley and rye-free

baking products long-term if the advice given in this Guide is followed as closely as possible. Your personal tolerance threshold is crucial
in this respect.

Breakfast

You have a very large selection of foods available
for breakfast. If you normally have a light breakfast,
low-FODMAP fruit is a good choice. You can never
go wrong with an egg for breakfast, either.

Bread is the only topic that requires your close attention. If you are very sensitive to bread, the only
safe way is to bake it yourself. The recipes in this
Guide are just a suggestion. You will either make
baking low-FODMAP bread your new hobby, or
you will simply have to reduce bread consumption.
If you find that a careful selection of bread and a
limited quantity gets you through the day without
symptoms, you have ample choice in spreads. Please
refer to the earlier section in this Guide to find out
how to make low-FODMAP bread. Specific recipes
are found at the end of this chapter.

As far as spreads are concerned, you are on the safe
side with butter, sausage, jam and hard cheese. Suitable warm drinks that you can choose for breakfast
are described in greater detail in the earlier sections
of this Guide. Refer to FODMAP tables for further
food choices. Generally, breakfast poses hardly any
problems in terms of food selection.

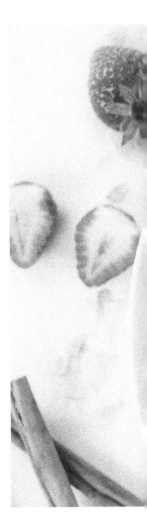

Light food that keeps you fuller, longer ...

Muesli with Blueberries, Kiwi and Tangerines

For 2 persons | ⏱ 10 min.

1 kiwi · 1 tangerine · 2 tbsp blueberries · 5 walnuts ·1 tbsp pumpkin seeds · 1 tbsp lime juice · 100 g oatmeal · 200 mL of lactose-free milk · 2 tbsp of maple sirup · 1 lactose-free yogurt

1   Peel kiwi and tangerine and cut them into suitable pieces. Add them to blueberries in a bowl and cover with walnuts, pumpkin seeds and lime juice.

2   Then add oat flakes, lactose-free milk, maple sirup and lactose-free yogurt, and mix everything.

Per serving: 452 kcal · 17 g protein · 16 g fat · 55 g carbohydrates

Buckwheat or quinoa flakes may be used instead of oat flakes. If you like your muesli very sweet, you may add maple sirup.

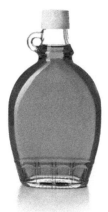

Maple Sirup

Maple sirup as a sweetener owes its roots to the North American Indigenous Peoples. The sirup gets its brownish color and typical aroma by the thickening of the naturally extracted juice from maple stems. If you do not fancy maple sirup, you can replace it with table sugar or sugar beet sirup.

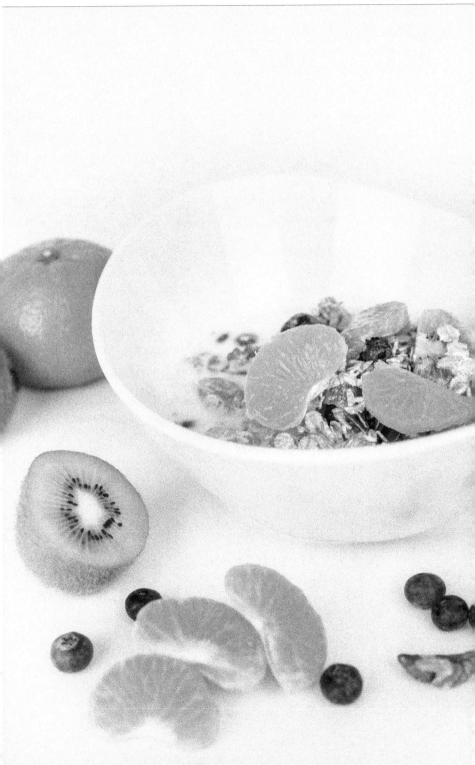

Refreshing and soothing ...

Pineapple-Mint-Drink

For 2 persons | ⏲ 5 min.

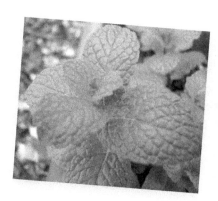

· ½ pineapple
· 1 bundle of fresh mint
· 2 tbsp of sugar
· 200 g of ice cubes
· 250 mL of orange juice

1   Peel the pineapple, remove the stalk and cut the pulp into small cubes. Pluck mint leaves from the stalks and set them aside for decoration.

2   Pour all the ingredients into an electric blender. Garnish with a few mint leaves and serve immediately after preparation.

Per serving 202 kcal · 2 g protein · 0 g fat · 44 g carbohydrates

It is also possible to mix a little bit of lactose-free cream into the drink, which makes the taste slightly different and the drink creamier.

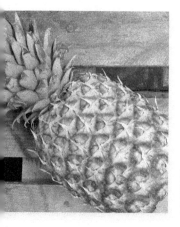

Mint and Pineapple

Mint and pineapple both have a positive effect on digestion, each in its own way. The enzyme bromelain in pineapple helps split proteins and thus facilitates their absorption. Pineapple also contains many minerals and vitamins. Mint has anti-spasmodic effects, and makes a refreshing drink.

Fruity, crunchy granola muesli in stock ...

Bluebeeries Granola

⏱ 10 min. + 30–45 min. baking time

400 g of oatmeal · 100 g of chopped almonds · 100 g of pumpkin seeds · 50 g of coconut chips · ¼ teaspoon salt · 1 coated tsp cinnamon · 1 pinch of ginger powder · 50 g of sugar · 3 tablespoons of vegetable oil · 5 tablespoons of maple syrup · blueberries · possibly lactose-free milk or lactose-free yogurt

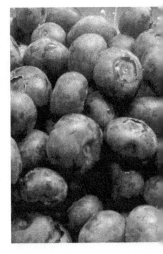

1   Take a large bowl and mix oatmeal, chopped almonds, pumpkin seeds, coconut chips and salt with a spoon. After stirring, add spices and sugar and mix thoroughly. Next, add oil and maple sirup and mix using your hands – use just enough oil and maple sirup to make oatmeal evenly moist.

2   Place a baking sheet on a baking tray and distribute the mixture evenly. Then bake granola for 15 minutes on the middle rack of an oven heated to 150 °C. Now turn the many small parts of granola with a fork and bake for another 15 minutes.

3   Depending on how crispy your want your granola, turn every 5 minutes and continue to bake until crispy enough. Usually, granola is ready after 2 to 3 turns when it adopts a light brown color.

4   Granola is best left to cool overnight in a dry place. It becomes crispy only upon drying.

5   Season it with blueberries, lactose-free milk or lactose-free yogurt just before serving. Instead of blueberries, you can also choose another low-FODMAP fruit, or eat granola without fruit, only with milk or yogurt.

Per 100 g: 464 kcal · 14 g of protein · 25 g of fat · 42 g of carbohydrates

Plenty of valuable protein ...

Strawberry Quinoa Breakfast

For 3 persons | ⏲ 20 min.

150 mL of rice milk · 1 teaspoon sugar · 200 g of quinoa · 1 pinch of salt · 200 g strawberries · 1 bundle of fresh mint · 30 g of almond slivers · ½ teaspoon of cinnamon · maple sirup, as desired

1   Bring 300 mL of water together with rice milk and sugar to boiling. If you do not have rice milk in stock, you can increase the amount of water instead. Add quinoa and a pinch of salt and simmer for 10–15 minutes at low temperature until the liquid has been absorbed.

2   In the meantime, cut strawberries into small pieces and mix with finely chopped mint leaves.

3   Remove quinoa from the heat and mix in almond slivers and cinnamon with a wooden spoon. Serve hot on small plates, seasoned with strawberries and the desired quantity of maple sirup.

Per serving 395 kcal · 12 g protein · 10 g fat · 60 g carbohydrates

Replace the maple-sirup with what you like best.

Quinoa

Quinoa is a „pseudocereal" commonly used in South America. Quinoa grains look like mustard or millet grains and can be used in many dishes. The use is similar to that of millet. Ground quinoa can be used as cereal flour and is particularly popular in patients with celiac disease as an alternative to cereals since this flour does not contain gluten. In addition, quinoa contains many essential amino acids and minerals.

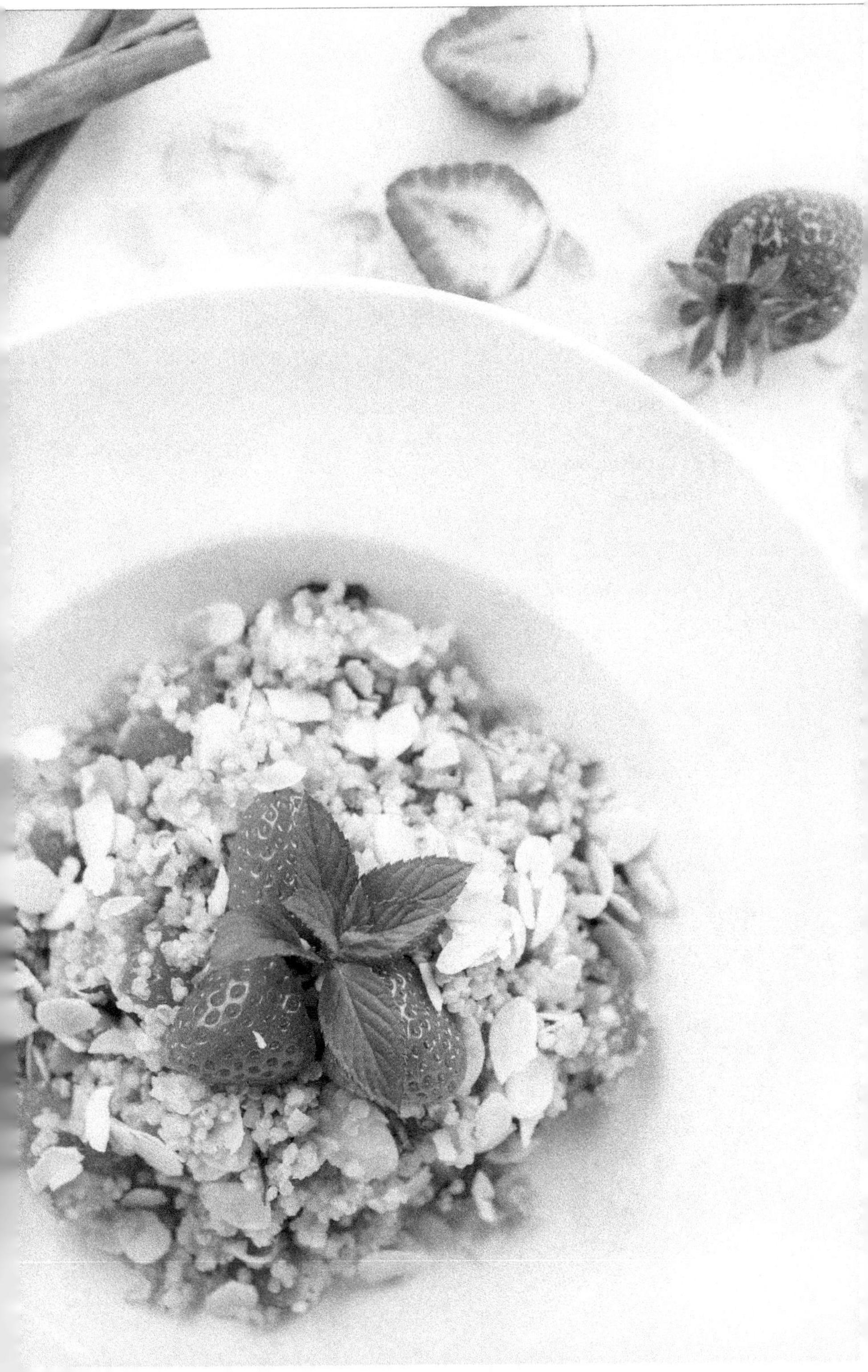

Savory with cheese and bacon ...

Breakfast Omelet

For 2 persons | ⏲ 15 min.

· 50 g of diced bacon
· 3 eggs
· Salt and black pepper
· 1 tomato
· 1 bell pepper
· Olive oil
· 50 g of grated pecorino
· Fresh chives

1   In a small pan, fry diced bacon until it becomes crispy.

2   Stir eggs in a mixing bowl with salt and pepper.

3   Cut tomato and paprika into very small pieces. Then mix tomato, pepper and bacon with eggs.

4   Place some olive oil in a pan, heat it and then add a scoop of the egg mixture into the pan, just enough to cover the bottom. Bake it golden brown on both sides like a pancake and sprinkle over pecorino cheese just before removing the pan from heat, allowing the cheese to melt.

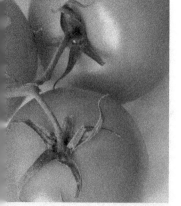

5   Fold the omelet and season it with finely chopped chives.

Per serving 511 kcal · 22 g protein · 45 g fat · 5 g carbohydrates

Creamy sweet temptation ...

Lemon Curd – Bread Spread

🕐 30 min.

3 large lemons, untreated · 250 g of powdered sugar · 1 packet of vanilla sugar · 3 eggs · 80 g of butter

1   First of all, run the lemon lightly across the grater so that just the bright yellow part of the rind is grated. Then squeeze the lemons and put the juice aside.

2   Stir the powdered and vanilla sugar and eggs vigorously in a mixing beaker.

3   Melt butter in a pot, add lemon juice, the egg-sugar mixture and the grated lemon peel. Stir everything and continue to cook at medium heat until the curd becomes creamy.

4   Fill the curd into screw-top jars and store in the refrigerator after it has cooled off. Lemon curd can be stored in a refrigerator for 10–14 days. But rest assured that once you taste it, it will not remain there that long!

Per 100 g 333 kcal · 4 g protein · 15 g fat · 46 g carbohydrates

Lemon Curd

Lemon curd is a very popular bread spread in the UK. It is in a mixture of sugar, eggs and lemons, which is used either as jam or for the refinement of baked goods. It has a very aromatic taste. Other curds, which consist mostly of coagulated milk and are widespread in Great Britain, have not yet established themselves on the European mainland.

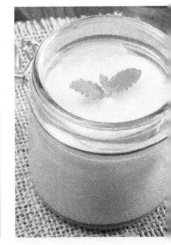

A breakfast classic reinvented ...

American Pancakes with Blueberries

For 4 persons | ⏱ 20 min.

240 g of rice flour · 80 g of starch · 3 tsp tapioca flour or soy flour ·
½ tsp xanthan · 1 packet of baking powder · 1 tsp sugar · ¼ tsp salt ·
1 knife tip of cinnamon · 2 eggs · 450 mL of lactose-free milk ·
3 tablespoons vegetable oil · 1 bowl of blueberries · maple sirup

1   First of all, whisk together all your dry ingredients in a mixing
bowl. Then mix in the eggs, lactose-free milk and oil. The batter
should be firm, but still roll out well in the pan. If it does not spread
well in the pan, add some milk to it.

2   Heat a little oil in a large skillet and pour batter into the pan using
a ladle. Spread the batter into a 8–10 cm circle, which is the typical
size of American pancakes.

3   At medium heat, bake one side, then turn and bake the other side.

4   Serve fresh, add blueberries and some maple sirup for sweetening.

Pro Portion 591 kcal · 17 g Eiweiß · 20 g Fett · 83 g Kohlenhydrate

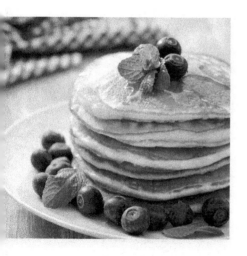

Tapioca

Tapioca is a starch extracted
from cassava root. It is na-
tive to Brazil. Tapioca flour
is used for similar things as
potato starch or corn starch.
In recent years, tapioca balls
habe been increasingly used
in sweets and bubble teas.

Healthy protein crispy fried ...

Savory Tofu Breakfast

For 3 persons | ⏱ 25 min.

150 g of solid tofu · pepper· 1 tbsp of soy sauce· garlic oil· 3 eggs · salt, pepper · fresh coriander (or chives)

1   Cut tofu into 3 thick slices, sprinkle with pepper and add some soy sauce. Let it soak in the soy sauce for 2–3 minutes and then slowly fry the tofu in a coated pan with some garlic oil on both sides at very low heat until it becomes crispy brown. To do this well, you must take your time because if you fry tofu too fast it will decompose. If you lack patience, then simply cut tofu into cubes and fry it at higher heat and with significantly more oil – deep-fry it, so to speak.

2   In another pan, prepare the three eggs sunny-side up and season with some pepper and salt.

3   Place the ready tofu on the breakfast plates, add a fried egg to each serving and decorate with a little fresh coriander.

Per serving 321 kcal · 16 g protein · 27 g fat · 3 g carbohydrates

Coriander

Coriander, also known as Arab parsley, is very similar to parsley, but it has a higher share of essential oils and therefore a more intense taste. Both the coriander seed and the fresh coriander herb can be used as a spice. The flavor of seeds differs from that of herbs.

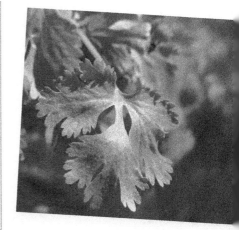

Creamy fruity and ready in no time ...

Kiwi-Smoothie

For 2 persons | ☽ 5 min.

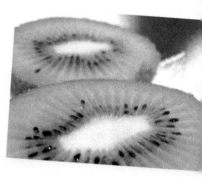

· **3 kiwis**
· **1 banana (firm)**
· **1 lime**

1   Peel kiwis and banana and cut them into pieces.

2   Put everything in a electric blender, add lime juice and mash it up.

3   Depending on the desired temperature and consistency, add 2–4 ice cubes and mash them in.

Per serving 94 kcal · 1 g protein · 1 g fat · 17 g carbohydrates

Spinach makes the difference ...

Popeye´s Orange-Smoothie

For 2 persons | ☽ 5 min.

2 oranges · 5 frozen strawberries · 1/4 avocado · 10 leaves of fresh spinach

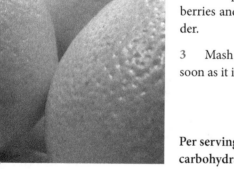

1   Peel oranges and cut them into pieces.

2   Add pulp of the oranges, avocado, strawberries and spinach leaves to an electric blender.

3   Mash for 30–60 seconds and drink it as soon as it is ready.

Per serving 120 kcal · 3 g protein · 3 g fat ·16 g carbohydrates

Breakfast eggs in a sophisticated manner ...

Poached Eggs

For 2 persons | ⏱ 20 min.

· 2 tablespoons of vinegar
· 4 large eggs
· Fresh chives
· Pepper, salt

1   Bring 1 ½ liter of water to boiling and add a small dash of vinegar. Bring the water to a light simmer over a medium heat.

2   Crack eggs one by one, and gently pour them into the simmering water. Leave the egg to cook for 2 ½–3 minutes at a slightly lower temperature.

3   Then remove the eggs from the water with a slotted spoon and drain onto kitchen paper. Now prepare the other eggs in the same way.

4   The preparation is somewhat easier if you boil the egg for 10 seconds in the shell, then crash the shell and pour the egg into the water.

5   The eggs can be kept warm in salt water at 30–40 degrees Celsius before they are served. They dry very quickly when they are not in the water.

6   Season the eggs with chopped fresh chives and coarsely ground pepper and add salt as desired.

Per serving 167 kcal · 14 g protein · 11 g fat · 2 g carbohydrates

If poached eggs do not turn out as desired, check if the eggs are indeed very fresh. A fresh egg in a bowl of water sinks to the bottom, while a not quite so fresh one floats.

Appetizers

You will rarely encounter difficulties with starters. All types of lettuce are low in FODMAPs. If you get accustomed to making salads with vinegar and oil, or with a simple vinaigrette, as I describe it several times in the recipe suggestions, then you already halfway there. A recipe for a very simple low-FODMAP vinaigrette can be found under „Field Salad With Chicken Breast".

Ready-to-use salad dressings should be avoided. You can easily make garlic oil or onion oil yourself.

Salads can be seasoned with low-FODMAP raw foods such as diced carrots or peppers.

It is a good idea to work with only a few ingredients when preparing appetizers because you can keep track of FODMAPs. The recipe suggestions for appetizers can also be used as a light main dish if a slightly larger quantity is used.

You can easily make garlic oil or onion oil yourself. Add 200 mL of olive oil to a small cooking pot, add finely cut garlic or onions, and simmer the oil at low temperature for 5–10 minutes with constant stirring, followed by brewing for 20 minutes.

Then let the oil cool down and pour it through a sieve into a small bottle. The oil can be kept in the refrigerator for 1-2 weeks.

Here you can transform duty into a hobby. By adding chopped fresh herbs, you can add a different flavor to the oil.

Crispy raw food ...

Kohlrabi & Carrot Salad with Fresh Mint

For 2 persons | ⏱ 15 min. + 30–60 min. rest period

· 2 kohlrabis
· 5 carrots
· Fresh mint
· 4 tbsp garlic oil
· 2 tbsp lemon juice
· Salt, pepper

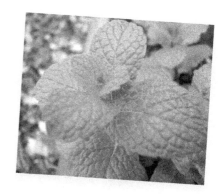

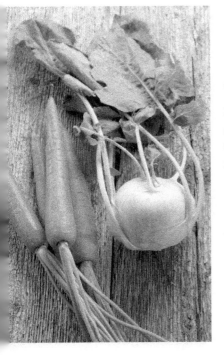

1   Peel kohlrabi and carrots first and then cut them into small strips.

2   Chop fresh mint and mix it with garlic oil, lemon juice and kohlrabi and carrot strips. Put some leaves of mint aside for decorating.

3   In a covered bowl, let it brew for 30–60 minutes.

4   Add salt and pepper to suit your taste, mix it in just before serving, and decorate with a few mint leaves.

Per serving: 317 kcal · 6 g protein · 15 g fat · 32 g carbohydrate

Green from the oven ...

Butterhead Lettuce in a Unique Way

Serves 2 persons | ⏲ 10 min. + 15–20 min. baking time

· 2 x butterhead lettuce
· Salt, pepper
· Fresh thyme
· 4 tbsp garlic oil
· 2 tbsp diced bacon

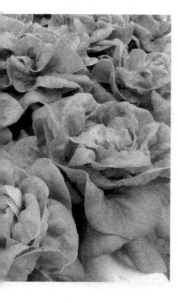

1   Cut the butterhead lettuce into halves and free them from the stalk. Place butterhead lettuce with the cut side facing up into a greased baking tray, season with salt, pepper and fresh thyme.

2   Add garlic oil. Cover the baking tray and place it on the middle rail of an oven heated to 170 degrees Celsius.

3   While the salad is in the oven, gently sauté the bacon bits in some garlic oil.

4   After 15–20 minutes, remove the lettuce and add bacon bits.

Per serving: 375 kcal · 4 g protein · 38 g fat · 3 g carbohydrate

This recipe brings a lot of variety to your kitchen because you can use other types of lettuce instead of butterhead lettuce. As each lettuce type tastes differently, your taste buds will not get bored. Just try curled lettuce with a nutty flavor!

The flavors of Southern fields on your table ...

Fried Eggplant

Serves 2 persons | ⏱ 25 min.

- · 1 large eggplant
- · 5 tbsp olive oil
- · Salt, pepper
- · 100 g of starch
- · 1 lemon, juice

1   Cut eggplant into 5-mm slices. Add salt and pepper, sprinkle with some lemon juice and oil, and allow to stand for about 10 minutes for the oil to get absorbed.

2   Place starch on a plate, put eggplant into it and then fry well in a pan on both sides.

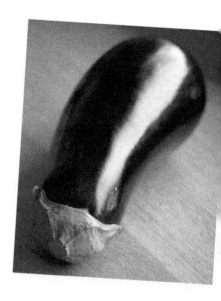

Per serving: 541 kcal · 2 g protein · 38 g fat · 48 g carbohydrates

The eggplant tastes a little more savory if it is additionally turned in egg after starch.

You can make eggplant even more delicious if you season the slices with some dark balsamic vinegar just before serving.

Spicy and delicious ...

Chard with Hot Feta Cheese

Serves 2 persons | ⏱ 30 min.

- · 2 tbsp of pine nuts
- · 2 pieces of feta cheese (about 200 g)
- · 6 leaves of chard
- · 2 tbsp of garlic oil
- · Salt
- · Freshly ground pepper

1   Roast pine nuts in a hot pan for 2–3 minutes until they turn light brown. Fold the two pieces of feta cheese in aluminum foil and bake them in a baking pan for 15–20 minutes in an oven pre-heated to 210 degrees Celsius.

2   Meanwhile, cut chard into broad strips, sauté them in garlic oil and steam for about 10 minutes with a little water. Season with a pinch of salt and plenty of freshly ground pepper.

3   Take the feta cheese slices from the oven, remove the foil and carefully place the slices on the chard.

Per serving: 521 kcal · 19 g protein · 47 g fat · 4 g carbohydrates

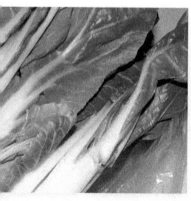
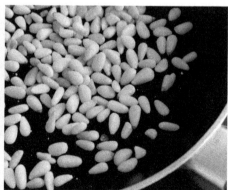

A special flavor combination ...

Parma Ham on Fennel & Dill Salad

Serves 3 persons | ⏱ 10 min.

· 2 fennel tubers
· 1 bunch of fresh dill
· 5 walnuts
· 1 tablespoon of mustard
· 5 tbsp of olive oil
· 5 tbsp of balsamic vinegar
· 1 teaspoon of sugar
· Salt, pepper
· 150 g of sliced Parma ham

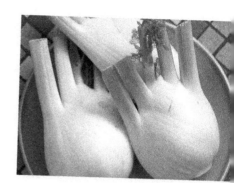

1   First off, wash the fennel, halve it and cut into 5-mm strips.

2   Chop the dill with a knife and cut the walnuts into coarse pieces.

3   Mix mustard, olive oil, vinegar, sugar, salt and pepper to make vinaigrette. Add a few tablespoons of water, depending on the desired texture of the vinaigrette.

4   Put fennel, dill and walnuts in a salad bowl and mix with the vinaigrette. Roll the ham slices individually and place them on top.

Pro Portion 307 kcal · 16 g Eiweiß · 24 g Fett · 7 g Kohlenhydrate

Simple low-FODMAP vinaigrette

Add 1 tbsp of mustard, 5 tbsp of balsamic vinegar, 5 tbsp of olive oil, 5 tbsp of water, a pinch of salt and a pinch of pepper to the vinaigrette.

You can season this simple vinaigrette with different freshly cut herbs to generate a variety of tastes.

A classic of Oriental cuisine ...

Hummus

Serves 3 persons | ⏱ 15 min.

1 glass chickpeas (about 330 g) · 100 g sesame paste (tahini) · 3 tbsp garlic oil · ½ lemon · ½ tsp ground cumin · salt · ¼ tsp peppers, hot · 1 red chilli pepper · 1 cucumber ·1 carrot

1   Pour the chick peas out of the glass through a sieve and discard the liquid. Then add chickpeas, sesame paste, garlic oil and 5 tbsp of water into a mixing bowl and mash it with a blender.

2   If you want to spice up the taste, you can add some pickled peppers; this way the hummus will adopt a more intense red color. Then stir in lemon juice and season with cumin and salt.

3   Spoon the hummus into a shallow serving dish and decorate it with some sesame or peppers or whole chickpeas.

4   Cut the bell peppers, cucumber and carrot into strips (about 10 cm long) and serve the hummus with the vegetable sticks.

Per serving: 507 kcal · 17 g protein · 35 g fat · 24 g carbohydrates

How to reduce FODMAPs

Chickpeas and sesame paste (Tahin) contain Oligosaccharides (the O in FODMAP). Oligosaccharides are water-soluble. By repeated soaking and throwing away the soaking water, the proportion of FODMAPs can be reduced. If you want to reduce the FODMAPs even more, you can replace half of the sesame paste with 75 g of lactose-free yogurt (1/2 cup).

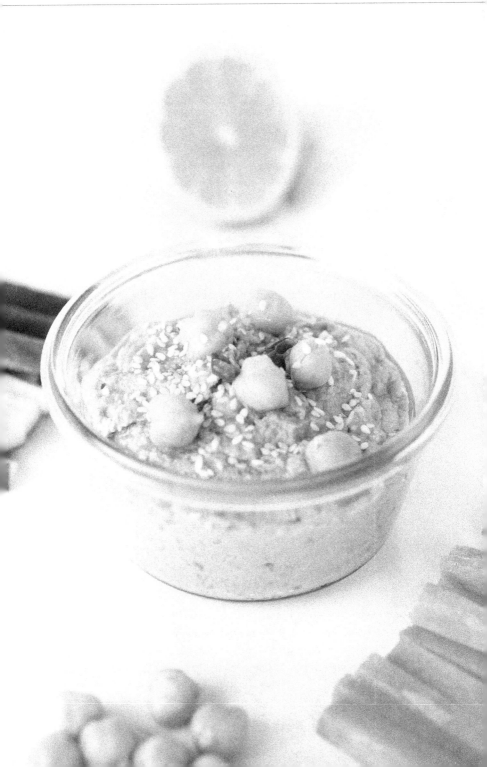

Quickly prepared and filling ...

Romaine Lettuce with Tuna

Serves 3 persons | ⏱ 10 min.

6 tbsp of olive oil · 6 tbsp of balsamic vinegar · 1 tbsp of sweet mustard · Salt, pepper · 1 Romaine lettuce · 1 tomato · ½ cucumber · 1 bunch of green onions (green parts) · 1 can of tuna in own juice · 3 hard-boiled eggs

1   Mix the oil, vinegar, mustard, 6 tbsp of water, salt and pepper to make the vinaigrette. The vinaigrette tastes even better when you add fresh herbs.

2   Wash the lettuce, tomato and cucumber, and cut them into small pieces. Cut the green parts of green onions into small pieces, and discard the white parts.

3   Put everything in a bowl and spread the tuna over it. Now add the vinaigrette and mix it.

4   Cut the hard-boiled eggs into quarters and place them on the salad.

5   The best is to enjoy the salad when the eggs are still warm, and if you take the Romaine lettuce from the refrigerator right before preparation.

Per serving: 273 kcal · 22 g protein · 17 g fat · 7 g carbohydrates

Balsamic vinegar contains fructose. If you want to substantially reduce the fructose content of the salad dressing, you can replace some of the balsamic vinegar with apple vinegar. This also applies to the fennel & dill salad on page 131, and the field salad with chicken breast on page 136.

You can taste the sun in it ...

Tomato Soup with Parmesan

Serves 3 persons | ⏲ 40 min.

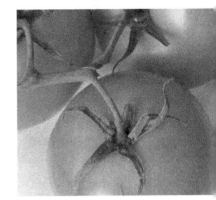

- · 1 kg tomatoes, finely cut
- · 500 mL of clear chicken broth
- · Fresh rosemary
- · 2 tbsp butter
- · 2 tbsp starch
- · 2 tbsp garlic oil
- · 1 spoonful of sea salt
- · 1–2 teaspoons of sugar
- · Salt, pepper
- · 100 g grated Parmesan cheese

1   Cut the tomatoes into small cubes. Alternatively, you can use diced tomatoes from the can (2 large cans).

2   Cook the small tomato cubes with the chicken broth and 2 sprigs of rosemary for ½ hour.

3   Remove the rosemary and pour the boiled tomatoes with the chicken broth once through a colander.

4   In a cooking pot, melt the butter and stir in the starch thoroughly so that no clumps remain.

5   Next, gradually stir the mashed tomatoes with the chicken broth with a whisk in the butter. Finally, season with garlic oil, salt, sugar and pepper.

6   Pour the soup into soup plates, sprinkle with a tbsp of Parmesan and let it melt for 1–2 minutes.

Per serving: 333 kcal · 8 g protein · 23 g fat · 21 g carbohydrates

Easily digestible indulgence ...

Field Salad with Chicken Breast

Serves 3 persons | ⏱ 20 min

· **6 tbsp olive oil**
· **6 tbsp balsamic vinegar (or alternatively apple vinegar)**
· **1 teaspoon mustard**
· **1 teaspoon soy sauce**
· **Pepper, salt**
· **1 bunch of chives**
· **500 g chicken breast**
· **200 g of field salad**
· **Freshly ground pepper**

1   Mix the oil, vinegar, mustard, soy sauce, salt, pepper, 6 tbsp of water and the chopped chives to make the vinaigrette. Add some extra water, which makes the vinaigrette more fluid and less spicy.

2   Pan-roast the chicken breast from both sides, season with salt and pepper and continue roasting until crispy and well done.

3   Cut the chicken breast into thin slices. If you like the chicken breast very crispy, you can sauté the slices again.

4   Wash the lettuce, spread it on the plates, and sprinkle the vinaigrette and some freshly ground pepper over it just before serving to keep the lettuce fresh. Now mix everything and place the chicken breast slices on top or at the side.

Per serving: 280 kcal · 40 g protein · 11 g fat · 3 g carbohydrates

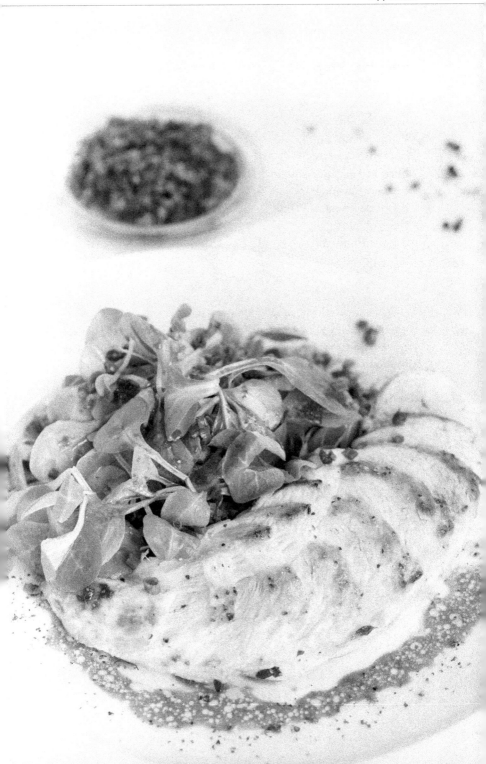

Rich with the flavors of autumn ...

Pumpkin Soup with Lemongrass and Coconut Milk

Serves 3 persons | ⏱ 45 min.

· 3 large potatoes
· 2 carrots
· 1 orange Hokkaido squash
· 2 stalks of lemongrass
· ¾ L of clear vegetable broth
· 3 tbsp of butter
· ½ L of coconut milk
· Salt, pepper
· Walnut oil

1   First off, peel the potatoes and carrots, and remove the seeds from the pumpkin. If you replace the orange Hokkaido squash with a different variety of squash, peel it before cutting. Sprinkle the lemongrass. Cut the pumpkin, potatoes and carrots into small pieces and cook together with the lemongrass for about 30 minutes in the broth until it turns soft.

2   Remove the lemongrass, and mash the vegetables with a blender. Then add butter and coconut milk, heat everything, but do not continue to boil.

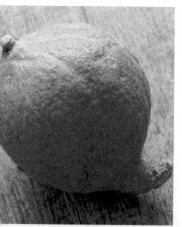

3   Finally, season with salt and pepper and dilute to the desired thickness with some vegetable broth.

4   Season the soup with some walnut oil.

Per serving: 543 kcal · 10 g protein · 23 g fat · 64 g carbohydrates

Indulgence with valuable fatty acids ...

Salmon Steak with Green Onions

Serves 2 persons | ⏱ 20 min + 4–5 hours in the fridge

300 g salmon · 4 green onions (green parts) · 1 bunch of coriander · ½ chilli (mild) · 2 tbsp olive oil · 1 tbsp garlic oil · ½ teaspoon ginger powder · 1/4 avocado · salt, pepper · 1 lime, juice

1 First cut the salmon into small cubes, measuring not more than 5 x 5 mm. It is easier to cut if you put salmon in the freezer half an hour before cutting it.

2 Then chop the green part of the green onions, coriander and chilli. Put some coriander aside for decorating.

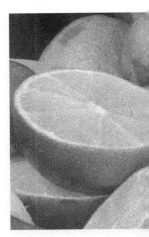

3 Mix the salmon, green onions, chilli peppers, oils, ginger and coriander with a fork. Finally season the tartare with salt and pepper.

4 Put in the refrigerator for 4–5 hours. Spread tartar on two plates.

5 Season the avocado with salt and pepper and place half of it on the plate next to the tartare. To decorate, add some fresh coriander leaves to the tartare. Just before serving, add some lime juice.

Per serving: 564 kcal · 31 g protein · 47 g fat · 4 g carbohydrates

Salmon tartare can be prepared in various ways. You can experiment a bit depending on what ingredients and spices you have in stock. For example, it tastes delicious with fennel instead of the green onions. Also, you can replace salmon with tuna filets.

Main dishes

As far as main dishes are concerned, you are free to do as you like. Almost. In the first 6–8 weeks of Phase 1 of your diet, it is essential to make the main dishes very simple and with few ingredients. You cannot go wrong with meat, fish or poultry. Do not use ready-made sauces for pasta; instead, season it only with salt, pepper and other herbs.

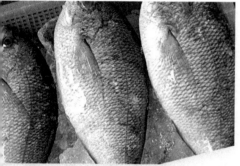

As for side dishes, you have plenty of choice if you refer to the table with low-FODMAP vegetables. It is easier to choose only one side dish at the beginning. If you want it a bit more elaborate and exciting, you will find below a few recipe suggestions for main dishes.

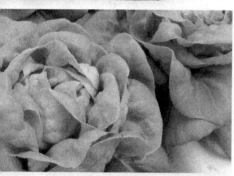

In Phase 2, as explained earlier in this Guide, you will gradually reintroduce individual foods into your diet until reaching your personal tolerance thresholds.

This means that you will gradually add foods rich in FODMAPs to your diet in phase 2, and learn how much you can tolerate and what quantity again leads to digestive complaints.

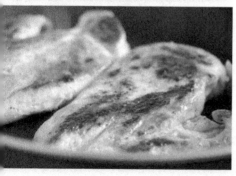

This tolerance threshold is very individual and a bit different for everyone. However, if you closely adhere to the food classification as ‚low in FODMAPs‘ and ‚high in FODMAPs‘, then you are on the safe side.

Much more than a culinary delight ...

Salmon with Colorful Rice

Serves 2 persons | ⏱ 25 min.

- · 150 g of rice
- · 1/2 corncob
- · 1 carrot
- · 1 stalk of broccoli
- · 1 red pepper
- · Salmon filets
- · Salt, pepper
- · 1 teaspoon of thyme

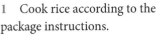

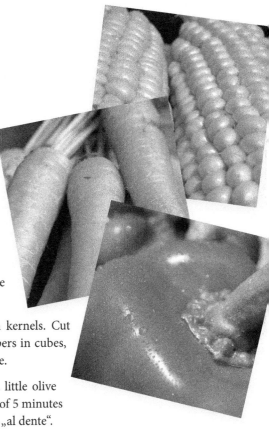

1 Cook rice according to the package instructions.

2 Meanwhile, cut the corn kernels. Cut the carrot, broccoli and peppers in cubes, approximately 1 x 1 cm in size.

3 Sauté the vegetables in a little olive oil and cook for a maximum of 5 minutes so that the vegetables remain „al dente".

4 While the vegetables are stewed, season the salmon with salt, pepper and thyme and fry in a pan at low temperature from both sides.

5 Finally, add the cooked rice to the vegetables and mix well.

Per serving: 915 kcal · 52 g protein · 45 g fat · 72 g carbohydrates

Soulfood for the whole family ...

Potato & Zucchini Gratin

Serves 4 persons | ⏱ 25 min. + 30 min. baking time

10 large potatoes · 3 large beef tomatoes · 2 zucchini · 3 eggs · 150 mL of lactose-free milk · 2 tablespoons oil · fresh rosemary · salt, pepper · nutmeg · 200 g grated hard cheese (Parmesan or Pecorino)

1   Precook the peeled potatoes 10–15 minutes and allow to cool.

2   Cut the tomatoes, zucchini and potatoes into thin slices. Grease a coverable casserole dish and add vegetables in layers, alternating tomatoes, zucchini and potatoes.

3   Mix the eggs thoroughly with milk, oil, chopped rosemary, salt and pepper, and pour over the vegetables. Now grate some nutmeg and finally sprinkle with cheese.

4   Bake the whole thing in the preheated oven on the middle rail for 25–30 minutes.

5   If your casserole is very full, then extend the baking time slightly. If you like a very crispy cheese crust, bake it without a lid on the top rail for the last 1–2 minutes.

Per serving: 798 kcal · 35 g protein · 28 g fat · 92 g carbohydrates

The potato & zucchini gratin makes an excellent main dish, but it is also a delicious side dish to a hearty beef filet or grilled fish. This dish becomes most delicious if you generously add fresh garden herbs. Thyme or rosemary are a must-try. The best thing is to add herbs just before serving.

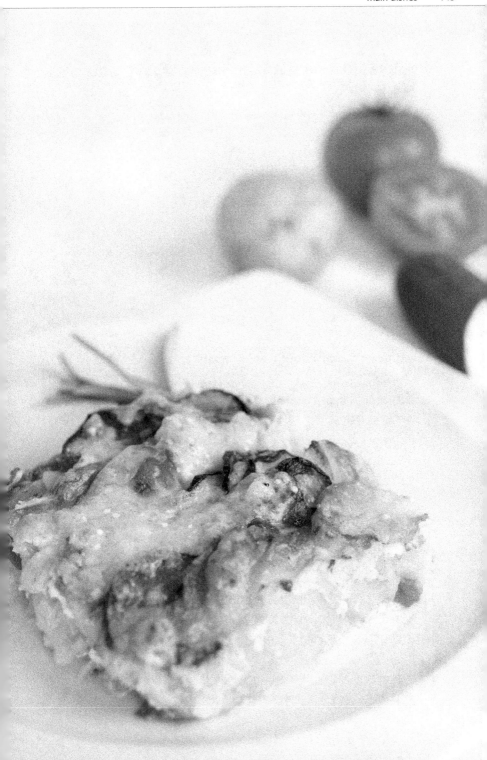

BBQ spits in exotic marinade …

Spicy Chicken Breast Spits with Pineapple

Serves 2 persons | ☉ 30 min. + 60 min. rest period

· 2 chicken breasts
· 2 tbsp of lactose-free yogurt
· 2 tbsp mustard
· 1 bunch of fresh coriander or parsley
· ½ tsp coriander seeds, cumin, chili (hot)
· Salt, pepper
· 4 tbsp garlic oil
· 1 pineapple
· 2 bell peppers (various colors)
· 6 cocktail tomatoes

1   Cut the chicken breasts into 3 x 2 cm pieces.

2   In a small bowl, make a marinade from lactose-free yogurt, mustard, finely chopped coriander, spices and oil. The yogurt does not have to be lactose-free, since only very little of it is used.

3   Place the marinade and the pieces of meat in a freezer bag, knead well and let it rest for an hour. You can also have the chicken breasts sit in a bowl, but the marinating is more intense in a freezing bag.

4   In the meantime, cut the pineapple and the peppers into 2 to 3 cm pieces.

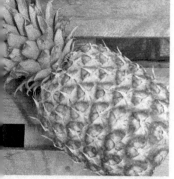

5   Thread the skewers, alternating peppers, pineapple, tomato and chicken. Chargrill for a minute, and then grill at medium heat for 10 minutes. Alternatively, the skewers can also be fried in a pan.

Per serving: 468 kcal · 34 g protein · 18 g fat · 36 g carbohydrates

Italian pasta – simply irresistible ...

Spaghetti Carbonara

Serves 4 persons | ⏲ 30 min.

500 g of spaghetti (buckwheat or quinoa) · 200 g of bacon, diced · 2 eggs · salt, pepper · 1 beaker of lactose-free cream · 100 g of grated Parmesan · 2 tbsp olive oil · fresh thyme

1   Cook the spaghetti according to package instructions.

2   Meanwhile, in a small pan, fry the diced bacon in olive oil until it is still somewhat glazed or very crispy, depending on your personal preference.

3   In a bowl, whisk the eggs with salt, pepper, cream and Parmesan cheese. You can also use 2 additional eggs instead of the cream, if you do not have any cream in the refrigerator.

4   Put the noodles back into the cooking pot after draining, add the bacon cubes and the egg mixture. Stir thoroughly with a wooden spoon and cover with a lid.

5   Actually, the residual heat of the noodles should be sufficient to cook the egg mixture. If not, simply heat again for one or two minutes at low temperature.

6   If you like, you can add some fresh thyme.

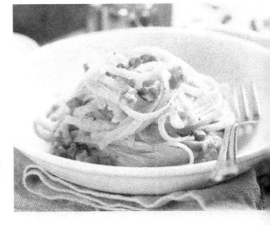

Per serving: 1064 kcal · 24 g protein · 63 g fat · 101 g carbohydrates

Provencal summer vegetables ...

Ratatouille

Serves 3 persons | ⏱ 50–60 min.

2 eggplants · 3 zucchini· 2 bell peppers (1 red, 1 green) · 5 tomatoes · 8 tablespoons olive oil · 2 large onions (for gentle roasting only) · fresh thyme · fresh rosemary · 1 bay leaf · 2 tablespoons garlic oil · salt, pepper

1   First cut the eggplant, zucchini, peppers and tomatoes into small, bite-size pieces. Cut the onions into thin slices.

2   In a large pot, heat the olive oil and add the onion rings. At low heat, gently roast the onions for 5 minutes, then remove them with a fork. Add the eggplant cubes, chargrill them briefly, and simmer for 5 minutes at low heat.

3   Then add the pepper cubes and the zucchini cubes and leave to simmer for about 15 minutes with the lid closed.

4   Finally, add the diced tomatoes, finely chopped herbs, the bay leaf and 3–4 tbsp. of water, and simmer the ratatouille for 20–30 minutes. Finally, season with garlic oil, salt and pepper.

Per serving: 555 kcal · 8 g protein · 50 g fat · 14 g carbohydrates

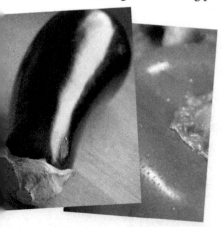

By the way, Ratatouille is delicious also when served cold. You can bake the leftovers in the oven the next day with hard cheese or mozzarella.

Culinary delights from the Orient ...

Peppers from the East

Serves 3 persons | ⌚ 40 min. + 40–50 min. of baking time

150 g rice · 4 large pointed peppers · 150 g ground meat · 200 g sheep's cheese (Feta) · 1 tbsp pine nuts · 1 bunch of coriander · ½ lemon, juice · 4 tbsp olive oil · 1 egg · salt, pepper

1 First, cook the rice according to the package instructions and allow to cool.

2 Cut the pointed peppers lengthwise in half and remove the seeds. Grease a casserole dish with some oil and place the peppers side by side.

3 Season the ground meat and sauté in a pan in oil, then allow to cool. Cut the sheep's cheese into small cubes, mix with the ground meat, rice, chopped pine nuts, chopped coriander, lemon juice, olive oil and eggs. Put a few coriander leaves aside for garnishing. Finally, season with some salt and pepper, and stuff the mass into the peppers.

4 The baking time in the oven pre-heated to 160 degrees is 40–50 minutes (and slightly longer in a non-preheated oven) .

5 Place a few coriander leaves on the peppers shortly before serving.

Per serving: 770 kcal · 30 g protein · 51 g fat · 46 g carbohydrates

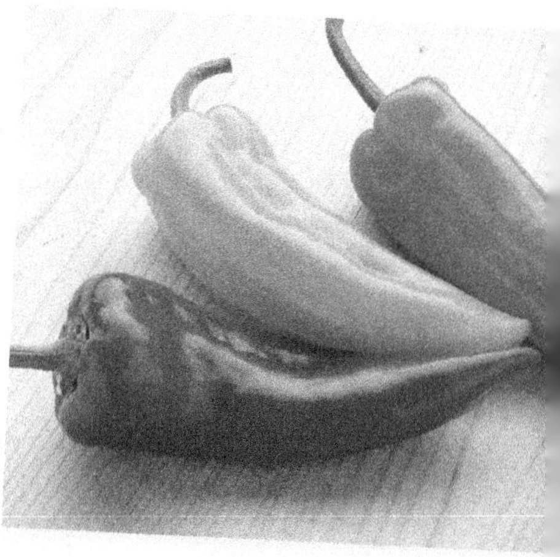

A mixture of fresh, chopped mint, dill and lactose-free yogurt is a delicious side item. Place it on the stuffed peppers just before serving.

Hearty casserole of ground meat and potatoes ...

Swiss Shepherd's Pie

Serves 4 persons | ⏱ 45 min. + 45–50 min. baking time

6 large potatoes · 40 g butter · 120 mL of lactose-free milk · salt, pepper · 300 g of ground beef · 300 g of ground lamb · 4 tbsp of olive oil · 3 carrots · 1 celery · 1 tomato · 1 sprig of rosemary · 1 sprig of thyme · 1 teaspoon of Worcestershire sauce (alternatively soy sauce) · 100 g grated Emmental cheese · pepper

1   First off, boil the peeled potatoes and make mashed potatoes with the addition of butter, milk and a pinch of salt and pepper.

2   In a high pan, fry the ground meat in olive oil well done.

3   Cut the carrots, celery and tomato into small slices or cubes.

4   Then gradually mix the vegetables and the spices into ground meat and simmer over a low heat for 30 minutes. Add small amounts of water if necessary.

5   Then remove the spice branches and season with salt and pepper. Put the vegetables and ground meat mixture into a greased baking dish. Spread the mashed potatoes onto it as a second layer, add a few drops of olive oil on top and bake the whole thing in a 180 degree oven for 45 minutes.

6   Just before the end of baking, add a thin layer of grated Emmental cheese and freshly ground pepper and place the casserole on top rail of the oven until the cheese is crispy.

7   Swiss Shepherd's Pie can be served as a main dish or as a side dish.

Per serving: 1037 kcal · 46 g protein · 59 g fat · 75 g carbohydrates

Cornmeal: Versatile, gluten-free and simply delicious ...

Polenta with Tomato & Cabbage & Vegetables

Serves 2 persons | ⏲ 40–45 min.

125 g cornmeal · ½ tsp salt · 25 g grated Parmesan cheese · 10 cocktail tomatoes · ¼ white cabbage · 1/2 celery · 2 tbsp olive oil · 1 tsp soy sauce · 1 tbsp balsamic vinegar · 8 green olives · 50 mL of lactose-free cream · salt, pepper · fresh basil or rosemary

1   Boil 500 mL of water with ½ teaspoon salt, then whisk cornmeal into the boiling water. Let polenta simmer at low heat for 15 minutes, then take off the heat and stir in Parmesan cheese using a wooden spoon. Allow to stand for 10–15 minutes and, voilà, your polenta is ready!

2   Cut the tomatoes in half, cut the white cabbage into strips and the celery in thin slices.

3   Heat the olive oil in a saucepan, sauté the white cabbage and the celery, and then stew for 3 minutes at low heat.

4   Add 5 tablespoons of water, soy sauce, balsamic vinegar, olives and tomatoes and stew for 3 more minutes. The olives can be added as desired – whole or quartered.

5   Finally, add the lactose-free cream and season with salt and pepper. For all purists out there, the cream can also be omitted, it is not a must!

6   Serve polenta and vegetables on a plate, and garnish with fresh basil leaves or fresh rosemary leaves.

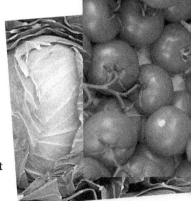

Per serving: 610 kcal · 13 g protein · 34 g fat · 58 g carbohydrates

A well-seasoned tossed in the frying pan ...

Tuna Steaks with Rice Noodles and Chard

Serves 4 persons | ⏲ 30–40 min.

- · 250 g of rice noodles
- · 1 bunch of chard
- · 1 carrot
- · 3 green onions (green part)
- · 4 tuna steaks
- · 3 tbsp garlic oil
- · 1 tablespoon lime juice
- · 2 tbsp wine vinegar
- · 1 tbsp soy sauce
- · 1 tbsp fish sauce
- · 1 tbsp brown sugar
- · Salt, pepper

1   Cook the rice noodles according to package instructions.

2   Cut the chard into medium-sized pieces, sauté in a pan in oil for a short time at high temperature and stew for 5 minutes at low temperature. Before serving, season the chard with some salt and pepper.

3   Cut the carrot and the green part of the green onions into thin strips.

4   Season the tuna steaks with salt and pepper and sauté in garlic oil on each side for 3–4 minutes. Add carrot and spring onion strips. Tuna steaks should be cooked medium rare. When they are ready, immediately remove them from the pan.

5   Drain the vegetables with lime juice, wine vinegar, soy sauce and fish sauce. Finally, stir in brown sugar, season with salt and pepper and add vegetable sauce over the rice noodles.

Per serving: 883 kcal · 53 g protein · 46 g fat · 62 g carbohydrates

Simply prepared and simply delicious ...

Spaghetti with Tomatoes and Mozzarella

Serves 4 persons | ☺ 30 min.

· **500 g of spaghetti (buckwheat or quinoa spaghetti)**
· **4 tomatoes**
· **200 g of mozzarella**
· **1 bunch of basil**
· **5 tbsp olive oil**
· **1 tbsp garlic oil**
· **Salt**
· **Freshly ground pepper**

1   Cook the rice noodles according to package instructions.

2   Cut the chard into medium-sized pieces, sauté in a pan in oil for a short time at high temperature and stew for 5 minutes at low temperature. Before serving, season the chard with some salt and pepper.

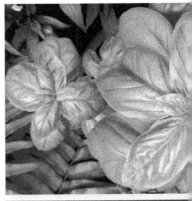

3   Cut the carrot and the green part of the green onions into thin strips.

4   Season the tuna steaks with salt and pepper and sauté in garlic oil on each side for 3–4 minutes. Add carrot and spring onion strips. Tuna steaks should be cooked medium rare. When they are ready, immediately remove them from the pan.

5   Drain the vegetables with lime juice, wine vinegar, soy sauce and fish sauce. Finally, stir in brown sugar, season with salt and pepper and add vegetable sauce over the rice noodles.

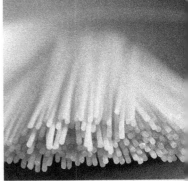

Per serving: 883 kcal · 53 g protein · 46 g fat · 62 g carbohydrates

Harmony of color and taste ...

Coalfish with Polenta Bites

Serves 2 persons | ⏲ 50 min.

125 g cornmeal · ½ tsp salt · nutmeg · 25 g grated Parmesan cheese · 2 salmon filets · salt, pepper · 1 tsp starch · 1 tablespoon oil · 1 lemon, juice

1   Boil 500 mL of water with ½ teaspoon salt, pour cornmeal into boiling water and finally whisk in some freshly grated nutmeg. Simmer over low heat for 15 minutes, take off the heat and allow to cool for 15 minutes.

2   Pour polenta on a baking sheet covered with baking paper, and allow to set and cool further.

3   When the polenta has cooled to room temperature, cut out squares or diamonds, 5–8 cm in size, place on a baking sheet and sprinkle with Parmesan.

4   Bake the polenta bites in the oven on the top rail for 5–10 minutes, until the Parmesan has melted and looks a little crispy.

5   Season the coalfish with salt and pepper, and turn in starch from both sides. Then, fry in a pan with oil, each side for 2–3 minutes, then remove and place on the plate and add a little lemon juice.

Per serving: 525 kcal · 49 g of protein · 14 g of fat · 49 g of carbohydrates

Coalfish with polenta bites tastes delicious when served with a side dish of zucchini or steamed red pepper, well seasoned with medium-hot chili peppers.

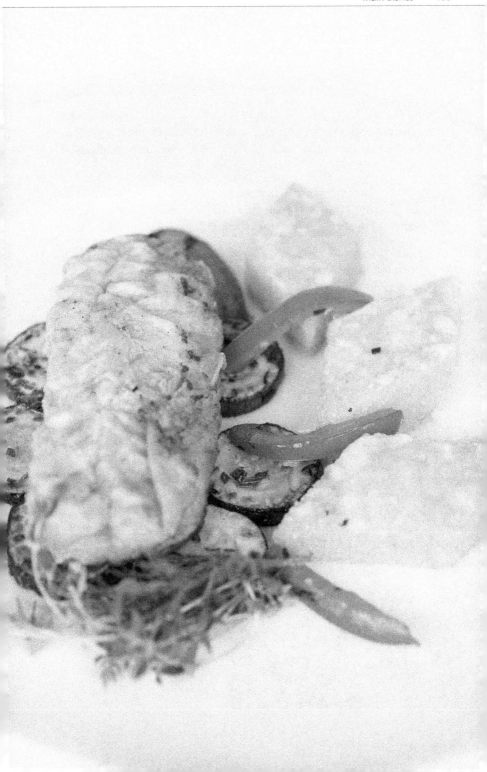

Desserts

You have to pay special attention when it comes to desserts since many desserts contain plenty of dairy products. Depending on your individual lactose tolerance, you can replace the dairy products in whole or in part with lactose-free products.

Lots of fructose also lurks in desserts, whether coming from the fruit itself or from the sweeteners used. You should also keep an eye on artificial sweeteners, which are mostly polyols.

And do not forget – many desserts contain recognizable or hidden cereals! Hence, you really need to pay attention to ingredients when eating desserts.

If you have not prepared the dessert yourself, just ask what it contains. Talking about a recipe is an uncomplicated and elegant way to break the ice and start a conversation.

It is best to avoid the ready-made desserts, unless you are able to fully grasp all ingredients and classify the food as low in FODMAPs. If in doubt, hands off!

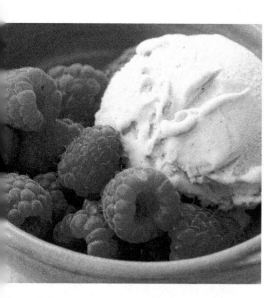

If you pay attention to the ingredients and keep the FODMAP content under control, you do not have to restrain yourself much when it comes to desserts.

A refreshing vitamin injection ...

Chilled Kiwi Soup

Serves 2 persons | ⏱ 5–10 min. + overnight in the fridge

- 5 kiwis
- 5 tbsp powdered sugar
- 1 packet of vanilla sugar
- 1 lime, juice
- 3 tbsp starch

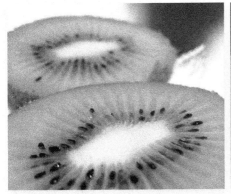 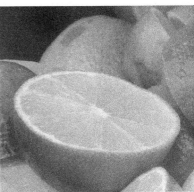

1   Peel the kiwis and cut them into small pieces. Leave half a kiwi intact. Pour the kiwis into a mixing bowl, add powder sugar, vanilla sugar and lime juice and purée everything with a blender.

2   Pour the kiwi mass into ½ L of water in a cooking pot and boil briefly.

3   Stir the starch with 4 teaspoons of lukewarm water in a cup. Take the boiling kiwi mass off heat, quickly whisk in the starch and boil again while stirring.

4   Put the mixture in a glass bowl and leave to stand in the refrigerator overnight.

5   Before serving, cut the remaining ½ kiwi into thin slices for garnishing.

Per serving 325 kcal · 1 g protein · 1 g fat · 73 g carbohydrates

The cult dessert from Italy loves it fruity ...

Coconut Panna Cotta with Kiwi

Serves 4 persons | ⏱ 30 min. + overnight in the fridge

5 leaves of gelatine · 200 mL of coconut milk · 300 mL of lactose-free cream · 50 g of sugar · 1 vanilla bean or 1 packet of vanilla sugar · 1 lemon, untreated · 2 kiwis · 1 tsp of brown sugar · cinnamon sticks, star anise or fresh mint for garnishing

1   Soften the gelatine leaves in lukewarm water.

2   Cut the vanilla bean in half lengthwise, scrape out the marrow and boil the bean and the marrow along with the coconut milk, cream, sugar and the finely grated lemon zest in a saucepan and simmer for about 5 minutes over low heat. Vanillla sugar can also be used instead of vanilla beans.

3   Remove the pot from the heat, let it cool for 1–2 minutes and then whisk the softened gelatin leaves into the hot cream.

4   If you do not want the lemon zest in the finished panna cotta, you can pour the hot cream through a sieve before adding gelatine. Next, fill the panna cotta into 4–6 ramekins (rinsed with cold water or greased with a little tasteless oil prior to filling). Keep it in a cold place overnight, or at least 4 hours.

5   Overturn the ramekin and let the panna cotta drop onto the plate. Sprinkle with a little brown sugar. Just before serving, peel the kiwis, cut them into thin slices and place around the overturned panna cotta. Add lemon juice to the kiwi.

Per serving: 413 kcal · 4 g protein · 34 g fat · 22 g carbohydrates

Run a dinner knife around the edge of the panna cotta to loosen it from the ramekin, and then place it briefly in warm water.

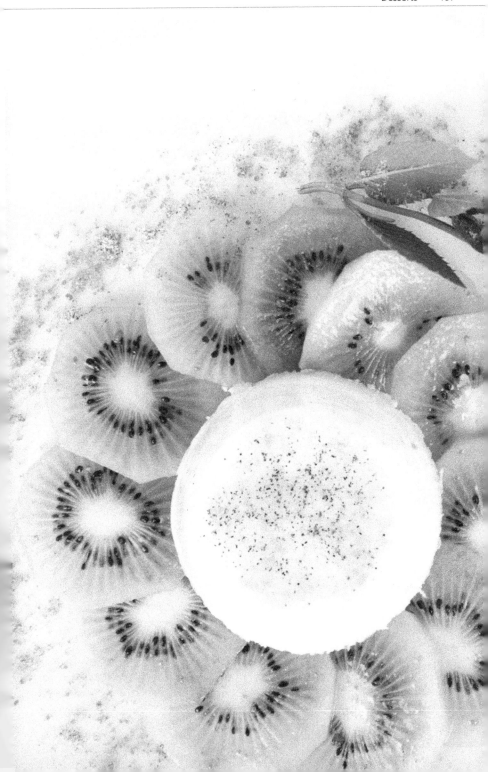

Vanilla and raspberry : The perfect couple ...

Bavarian Cream with Hot Raspberries

Serves 4 persons | ⏱ 20 min. + overnight in the fridge

5 leaves of gelatine · 300 mL of lactose-free milk · 200 mL of lactose-free cream · 1 vanilla bean · 4 egg yolks · 80 g of sugar

For hot raspberries:
250 g of frozen raspberries · 2 tbsp of sugar

1   Soften the gelatine leaves in lukewarm water.

2   Cut the vanilla bean in half lengthwise, scrape out the marrow and warm the bean and the marrow along with milk and cream in a pot. Simmer for about 5 minutes at low heat, while stirring continuously, but do not boil.

3   In the meantime, whisk the egg yolk with sugar in a beaker.

4   Remove the vanilla bean and slowly add the egg yolk - sugar mixture to the hot milk – cream mixture with constant stirring. Squeeze out the gelatine leaves, and continue stirring until the cream thickens.

5   Then pour the cream into small bowls and put them in the refrigerator overnight.

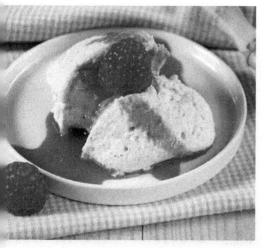

6   Warm up the raspberries along with sugar and 4–6 tablespoons of water in a small saucepan and spread over the Bavarian cream.

Per serving: 421 kcal · 10 g protein · 25 g fat · 36 g carbohydrates

A delicious dessert for the whole family ...

Pineapple & Strawberry Jelly with Vanilla Sauce

Serves 4 persons | ⏲ 25 min. + overnight in the fridge

· 5 leaves of gelatin
· 1 medium-sized can of pineapple (about 350 g of pineapple and 200 mL of juice)
· 200 mL of orange juice
· 4 tbsp of sugar
· 2 cups of strawberries (about 400 g)

For vanilla sauce:
· 1 heaping tbsp of starch
· 2 tbsp of sugar
· 3 egg yolks
· 350 mL of lactose-free milk
· 1 vanilla bean or 1 packet of vanilla sugar

1   Soften the gelatine leaves in lukewarm water.

2   In a pot, bring the pineapple juice, orange juice and sugar briefly to a boil. Then add the finely cut strawberries and pineapple and simmer for 15 minutes at low heat until the fruits become soft.

3   Allow the fruit mixture to cool a little, then whisk in the gelatine leaves until they dissolve. Put the jelly in a large glass bowl and refrigerate overnight.

4   To make vanilla sauce, thoroughly mix the starch, sugar and egg yolk. In a small saucepan, bring the milk with the marrow of the vanilla bean and the halved bean to a boil, and cook for 15 minutes at low heat. If you do not have a vanilla bean, you can use vanilla sugar instead.

5   Next, remove the vanilla bean. Now whisk in the eggyolk mixture and continue stirring at low heat until the sauce becomes creamy. Do not boil after adding the egg yolk.

Per serving: 375 kcal · 10 g protein · 9 g fat · 59 g carbohydrates

Wickedly delicious chocolate delight ...

Bittersweet Chocolate Mousse

Serves 4 persons | ⏲ 25 min. + 3–4 hours in the fridge

200 g dark bittersweet chocolate, cocoa content at least 70 % · 50 g butter · 200 mL of lactose-free cream · 3 eggs · 2 tbsp sugar · 1 tsp cocoa · 1 packet of vanilla sugar · 1 tbsp slivered almonds · fresh mint · some strawberries for garnishing

1   Break the chocolate into small pieces and melt together with butter in a water bath. When the chocolate has completely melted, stir in the cream.

2   In a mixing bowl, mix the egg yolk with sugar, vanilla sugar and cocoa to generate a creamy mass and then fold the melted chocolate into the mixture.

3   Beat the egg whites and fold them into the mousse.

4   Pour the mousse into small bowls and place in the refrigerator for 3 to 4 hours.

5   Sprinkle with slivered almonds shortly before serving, and garnish with a slice of strawberry and a mint leaf.

Per serving: 648 kcal · 11 g protein · 51 g fat · 32 g carbohydrates

Chocolate

Cocoa contained in the chocolate is low in FODMAPs. Only the milk components and the sugar used in chocolate make chocolate high in FODMAPs. Therefore, dark chocolate with a high cocoa content is better tolerated than milk chocolate. Due to the high fat content, chocolate should be enjoyed in moderation.

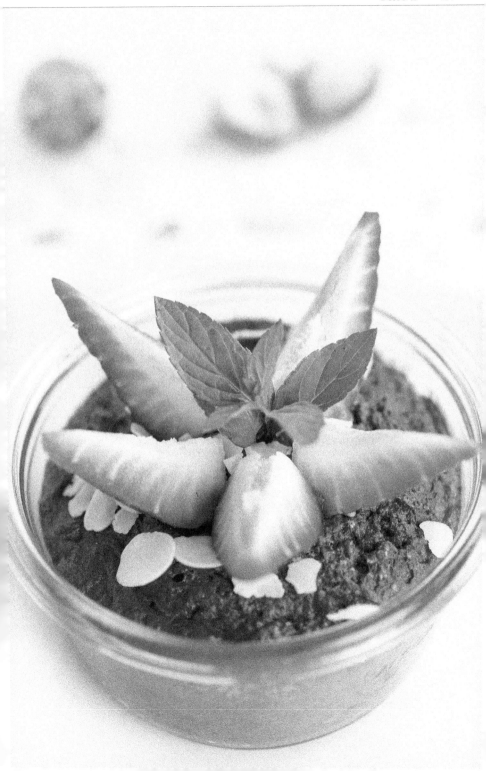

Wholesome dessert without gluten ...

Millet & Banana & Kiwi Dessert

Serves 4 persons | ⏱ 60 min.

· 240 g of millet
· 2 bananas (firm)
· 3 tsp sugar
· ¼ tsp ground cardamom
· 20 g of butter
· 2 tsp of sugar
· ½ teaspoon of cinnamon
· 2 kiwis

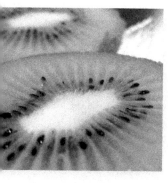
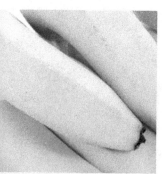

1   Soak millet in 300–350 mL of water for 30 minutes, then slowly heat it until it simmers. Half of the water can be replaced by lactose-free milk, which renders the dessert somewhat creamier.

2   Grate a banana with a fork and add to the millet together with sugar, cardamom and butter. Allow the mixture to simmer for 30 minutes and then heat it for a little longer or add some water, depending on the desired texture.

3   While the millet simmers, make a cinnamon-sugar mixture from sugar and cinnamon.

4   Cut the second banana into slices and the kiwi into small pieces.

5   Shortly before serving, add banana and kiwi into the millet gruel and, depending on your taste, sprinkle the individual portions with the cinnamon-sugar mixture.

Per serving: 342 kcal · 7 g protein · 7 g fat · 60 g carbohydrates

Sweet cornmeal tastes delicious as well ...

Polenta Cake with Fresh Strawberries

⏱ 30 min. + 50 min. baking time

· **200 g of butter**
· **200 g of powdered sugar**
· **100 g of cornmeal**
· **½ pack of baking soda**
· **200 g grated hazelnuts**
· **3 eggs**
· **2 limes, untreated**
· **250 g of strawberries**
· **5 tablespoons of maple sirup**

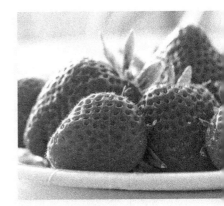

1   Mix the butter and powdered sugar with a fork or a hand mixer. Add cornmeal, baking powder and nuts, and then stir in 3 eggs and the grated lime zest.

2   Wash the strawberries and cut them in quarters. Mix them with lime juice and maple sirup, then stir the strawberries into the polenta dough.

3   Place baking paper on a baking tray and pour in the dough.

4   Bake the cake at 180 degrees in the preheated oven for 40–50 minutes. Using a thin metal stick or a toothpick, test whether or not the dough is still sticky. If this is the case, bake for another 5 minutes and repeat the test.

Per piece (⅛): 554 kcal · 7 g protein · 38 g fat · 46 g carbohydrates

A sweet meringue kiss ...

Raspberry Cream Meringue

Serves 4 persons | ⏱ 10 min. + allow to stand for 1 hour at room temperature

· 1 packet of meringue (lactose-free)
· 500 g of frozen raspberries
· 400 mL of lactose-free cream
· 1 packet of vanilla sugar

1   First of all, crush the meringues and place them in a glass bowl.

2   Then spread the frozen raspberries and the vanilla sugar over them, and put the whipped cream on top. Let it rest for an hour so that the raspberries can defrost.

Per serving: 448 kcal · 6 g protein · 30 g fat · 33 g carbohydrates

Meringues are low in FODMAPs, but unfortunately very high-calorie with about 400 kcal / 100 g. However, meringues are very suitable for the low-FODMAP diet as a dessert or snack, and are very versatile.

Homemade meringues: Beat 3 eggs and add a few drops of lemon juice. Then carefully fold in 150 g of sugar and ensure that the egg-white does not collapse. Cover a baking tray with baking paper and place the egg whites in 6–8 portions. Bake in the preheated oven at 110–120 degrees Celsius for 60 minutes, then leave to stand for an hour while the oven is switched off and open. The meringues should be crisp and light, but not browned.

Meringues taste delicious without any additions as well, but why not try them with lemon curd?!

Creamy and fruity without many calories ...

Kiwi & Orange & Curd Dessert

Serves 2 persons | ⏱ 10 min.

- · 2 kiwis
- · 1 orange
- · 1 cup of lactose-free yogurt (approx. 150 g)
- · 1 cup of lactose-free low-fat curd (approx. 150 g)
- · 1 packet of vanilla sugar
- · 1 heaping tbsp sugar
- · ½ lemon, juice

1   Peel the kiwi and orange and cut into small pieces.

2   In a bowl, mix the curd and yogurt thoroughly, and then add va-nilla sugar, sugar and lemon juice. Finally, mix in the fruit, pour into small bowls and serve chilled.

Per serving: 221 kcal · 16 g protein · 3 g fat · 29 g carbohydrates

Curd tastes delicious if you add 1 tablespoon of rum. Caution: Curd is then not suitable for children.

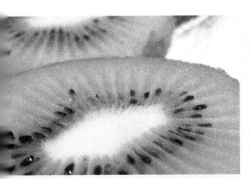
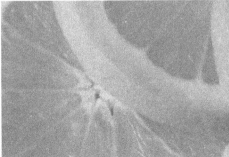

Enticing notes of coffee and sweet flavor – A delightful combination ...

Mocha Hazelnut Cream

Serves 4 persons | ◷ 120 min. + 4 hours in the fridge

- **450 mL of rice milk**
- **1 pinch of salt**
- **50 mL of coffee (strong)**
- **1 tbsp grated hazelnuts**
- **4 tbsp of sugar**
- **1 packet of vanilla sugar**
- **60 g of starch**

1 Bring the rice milk with a pinch of salt, coffee, grated hazelnuts, sugar and vanilla sugar to a boil in a pot.

2 Meanwhile, mix starch with 4 tbsp of cold rice milk. As soon as the rice starts boiling, take the pot off the heat, whisk in the starch and then boil the rice milk again for 1–2 minutes until it becomes somewhat creamy.

3 Pour the cream into serving dishes and refrigerate for at least 4 hours.

Per serving: 205 kcal · 1 g protein · 4 g fat · 42 g carbohydrates

Milk substitutes

Soy milk, rice milk, almond milk, oat milk and other milk substitutes have little in common with cow's milk except color. These are foods that are produced in a variety of ways and are very different, depending on the manufacturer, so that making a general statement about their FODMAP content is rather difficult. When reviewing the ingredients, you should make sure that no ingredients high in FODMAPs have been added. Soy milk from soybeans and oat milk are high in FODMAPs (oligosaccharides). Rice milk and almond milk, on the other hand, have a lower FODMAP content.

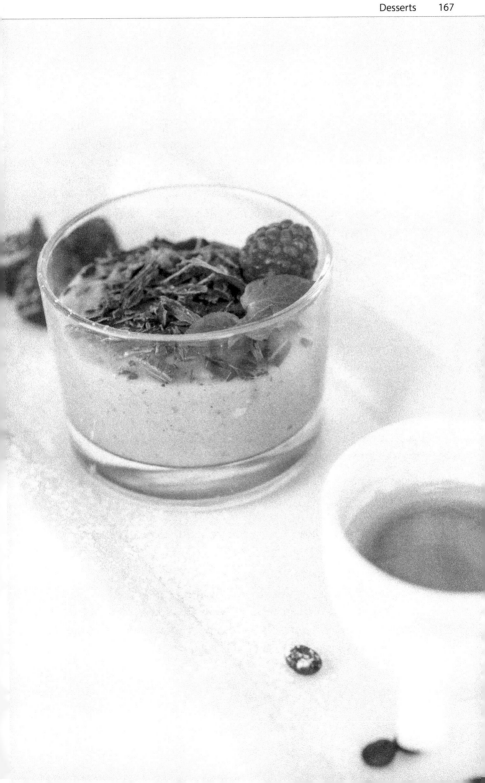

Bread recipes

Baking bread at home, especially with low-FODMAP flour, is no job for a beginner. Conventional wheat bread cannot be made with the substitute flour such as rice flour, soy flour, starch, etc. The dough

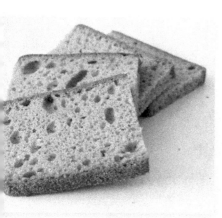

does not rise adequately, the texture of the breads is something one must get used to, and the crusts do not always look nice.

All these disadvantages should be compensated for by the taste and joy of your own creativity. Do not be discouraged by a failed bread. At the beginning stage, try to deviate from the recipes only in small steps so that you can track which change led to the change in taste, shape and appearance of your bread.

If you continuously fail, or if you find the process too cumbersome, you can resort to using the available wheat-free bread baking mixtures for the oven or for the baking machine.

Since you need not adopt a completely wheat-free diet, you can also choose the recipes of your bread-baking machine. You can replace half of the amount of the wheat flour with a mixture of 2 parts of rice flour, 1 part of soy flour, 1 part of starch and 1–2 tsp of xanthan per 500 g.

You can regulate the firmness of the bread with the amount of xanthan gun. If you like it more firm, take 2 teaspoons of xanthan gum per 500 g of flour. If you prefer it softer and looser, take 1 teaspoon of xanthan per 500 g of flour. The same applies to the alternative bread products such as carob bean gum and guar gum.

All home-baked loaves are kept at room temperature for three days; thereafter, however, bread with a high rice flour share will dry out very quickly.

Carob bean gum (E410)

Carob bean gum (E410) is a thickener and binder obtained from the seeds of the carob tree. Since humans cannot digest carob bean gum, it is often used in industrially processed foods. Carob bean gum replaces gluten in gluten-free baked goods.

Guar gum (E412)

Guar gum (E412) is a thickening and emulsifying agent obtained from the guar bean. Just as carob bean gum, guar gum is not digestible for humans. Guar gum is used in industrially processed foods and in cosmetic products. Guar gum also replaces gluten in gluten-free baked goods, its adhesiveness however, is lower than that of xanthan gum

Xanthan gum (E415)

Xanthan gum (E415) is a thickening and gelling agent produced by bacteria. Since humans cannot digest xanthan gum, it is used in many foods and cosmetic products. The thickening ability of xanthan gum is somewhat greater than that of guar gum and carob bean gum.

Flour trio for your favorite mixture ...

Low-FODMAP Bread

⏱ 20 min. preparation + 60 min. rise time + 60 min. baking time

· 3 eggwhites
· 200 g of tapioca flour
· 300 g of wheat flour
· 250 g of rice flour
· 1 tsp salt
· 1 packet of baking powder
· 1 tbsp xanthan gum
· 250 mL of water
· 1 packet of dry yeast
· 2 heaping tbsp of sugar
· 20 g of butter

1   Stir the egg whites stiff in a mixing beaker.

2   In a large bowl, mix the flours with salt, baking powder and xanthan gum.

3   Then add water, yeast and sugar and mix well with a hand mixer.

4   When everything is evenly mixed, add the soft butter and continue stirring. Finally, fold in the stiff protein at a low stirring speed.

5   Place baking paper on the baking tray and pour in the dough. Let the dough rise in a warm place for an hour.

6   When the dough has risen, bake the bread at 210 degrees Celsius in the preheated oven for about 60 minutes. Just before the end of the baking period, pierce the bread with a thin metal stick to check whether it already done. The baking time can be adapted according to the desired crust color and crust firmness.

Gluten-free, rich in protein, healthy ...

Buckwheat Bread

⏲ 20 min. preparation + 60 min. rise time + 60 min. baking time

700 g buckwheat flour · 50 g potato starch · 1 tsp salt · 1 tsp sugar · 1 packet baking powder · ½ bag dry yeast · 500 mL of water · 3 tbsp vegetable oil · 1 tsp sesame

1   First of all, place all dry ingredients in a large mixing bowl and mix with a spoon. Then add water and vegetable oil and mix with a stirrer until a tough dough is formed.

2   The dough should be easily loosened from the edge of the bowl. Add some more water or a little more flour as required. Leave the dough in a warm place for 30–60 minutes.

3   Grease a bread baking dish or coat with baking paper and pour in the dough. The bread is then baked in the preheated oven at 200 degrees Celsius for 60 minutes.

4   Brush the surface of the dough with some salty water just before the end of the baking period and sprinkle with sesame seeds.

5   Just before the end of the baking period, pierce the bread with a thin metal stick to check whether it already done. The baking time can be adapted according to the desired crust color and crust firmness.

Buckwheat

Unlike the name indicates, buckwheat is not a cereal. Buckwheat is a knotweed plant and, like quinoa and amaranth, belongs to pseudo-cereals. Buckwheat contains no gluten and can replace grain when baking. Buckwheat tastes herb-nutty and a lot of valuable protein. It is traditionally used in Russian blinis, a kind of pancake.

The gluten-free power pack ...

Oat Bread

🕐 15 min. preparation + 60 min. rise time + 50 min. baking time

100 g oatmeal · 500 g oat flour· 450 mL of lactose-free milk · ½ tsp bread spice · 1 heaping tsp of salt · 1 packet dry yeast · 1 tbsp maple sirup · 2 tbsp of steel-cut oats

1   Mix all the ingredients in a mixing bowl to make the dough and leave to rest for an hour in a warm place.

2   Place a baking paper on a baking tray and shape the dough into a round, flat bread. Now let the bread rest for another hour in a warm place. If desired, sprinkle some steel-cut oats over it and press gently. For more crust, cut the dough as in the picture (cross-shaped).

3   Before and during baking, sprinkle/brush the bread loaf a few times with water. Bake the bread for about 50 minutes in a non-pre-heated oven at 200 degrees Celsius. Place a suitable oven-proof bowl of water in the oven to prevent the bread from drying out.

4   Just before the end of the baking period, pierce the bread with a thin metal stick to check whether it is already done. If you prefer a darker crust, bake the last 5–10 minutes on the top rail, otherwise on the middle or the bottom rail.

Oats

Oats are the healthiest of the classic cereals. And unlike wheat, rye and barley, oat contains only a small amount of gluten. The iron content of the savory panicle cereal is considerable, and one can further increase its bioavailability with vitamin C. The high content of calcium and B vitamins is good for hair, skin and our nervous system.

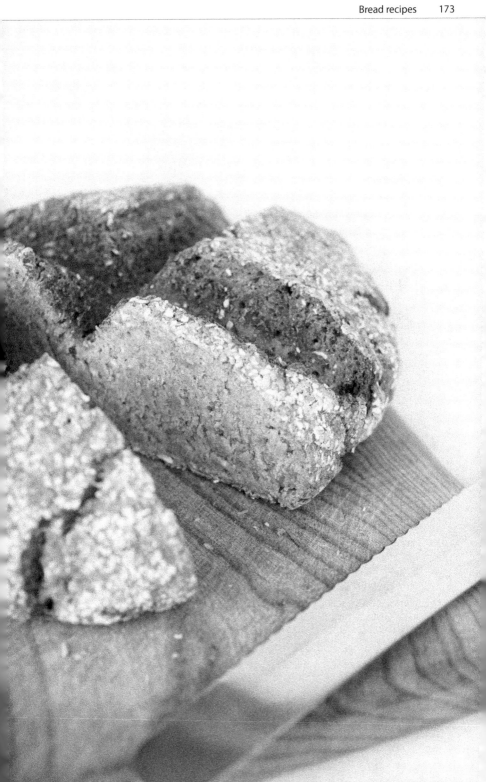

A delicious taste combination ...

Buckwheat Corn Bread

🕑 15 min. preparation + 60 min. rise time + 90 min. baking time

· 300 g of buckwheat flour
· 350 g of corn flour
· 50 g of starch
· 1 tsp carob bean gum
· ½ tsp coriander
· 5 tbsp of sunflower seeds
· 2 packs of baking soda
· 2 tsp salt
· 3 tbsp of maple sirup
· 750 mL of sparkling water

1   In a mixing bowl, first mix the buckwheat flour, corn flour, starch, carob bean gum, coriander, sunflower seeds, baking powder and salt with a spoon.

2   Then stir in the maple sirup and sparkling water with a hand mixer at the lowest level. Gently stir in the sparkling water since the carbon dioxide is used as a baking agent and escapes when stirring is too vigorous.

3   Place a baking paper on a baking tray and pour in the dough. Preheat the oven to 150 degrees Celsius and bake the bread for 90 minutes.

4   Just before the end of the baking period, pierce the bread with a thin metal stick to check whether it is already done. The baking time can be adjusted according to the desired crust color and thickness.

5   The taste of this bread can be varied by adding various bread spices or crushed grains. Bread spices usually contain cumin, aniseed and fennel and are available in health food stores.

Recipes for the bread baking machine

Bread baking machines are available in various sizes. The recipe suggestions are for baking machines with a baking bowl of 750–1000 g. If your baking machine has a different size, please adjust the quantities accordingly.

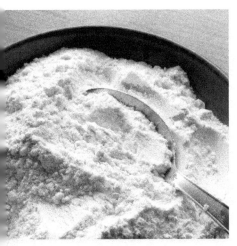

Each bread baking machine has its own programs to choose from. Since these programs differ, each recipe proposes a particular program. However, it may be necessary to use a different program depending on the baking result, or to lengthen or shorten the baking time using the browning settings.

Depending on your personal tolerance for cereals, you can use the bread recipes of your machine and replace 1/3 to ½ of the flour with cereal-free flours, which are described earlier in this Guide, or with gluten-free substitute flour, which you can buy in any health food store.

Your low-FODMAP breads will taste much better if you turn bread baking into your hobby and dive into the world of sour dough. All that is required is enough interest, will and time to get acquainted with the matter. Rest assured that you will quickly become a sour dough expert !

Perfect not solely in bubble tea ...

Tapioca Rice Bread

🕐 Baking time approx. 3 ½ hours in a bread baking machine

250 mL of lactose-free milk · 150 mL of water · 2 tablespoons of maple sirup· 2 tbsp olive oil · 1 tsp vinegar · 1 egg · 300 g of rice flour · 170 g potato starch · 60 g tapioca flour · 1 tsp xanthan gum · 1 bag of dry yeast · ½ tsp of salt

1   First off, add the liquid ingredients in the bread baking machine. Then add the dry ingredients.

2   For baking, choose a full-grain bread program with a total time of approx. 3 ½ hours.

A neutral mixture perfect for seasoning ...

Rice Soy Bread

🕐 Baking time approx. 3 hours in a bread baking machine

360 mL of water · 2 tsp maple sirup · 1 tsp olive oil · 200 g rice flour · 200 g corn starch · 100 g soy flour · 1 tsp xanthan gum · 1 packet dry yeast · 1 packet baking powder · ½ tsp bread spice · 1 tsp salt

1   First off, add the liquid ingredients in the bread baking machines. Then add the dry ingredients.

2   For baking, choose a standard or a white-bread program with a total time of approx. 3 hours.

3   Give creativity free reign with this bread! Try adding oregano or sesame instead of the bread spice.

Juicy and aromatic ...

Buckwheat Millet Bread

🕐 Baking time approx. 3 hours in a bread baking machine

320 mL of water · 200 g buckwheat flour · 100 g millet flour · 30 g dry sour dough · 1 packet dry yeast · ½ tsp bread spice · ½ tsp salt

1   Pour water into the bread baking machine. Mix all the dry ingredients in a bowl and place in the bread baking machine.

2   Bake the bread in the baking machine with a 3-hour white-bread program (usually program 1 or 2).

Hard to believe: without wheat ...

Wheat-free White Bread

🕐 Baking time approx. 3 hours in a bread baking machine

350 mL of water · 2 tbsp olive oil · 300 g rice flour · 80 g potato starch · 80 g corn starch · 40 g tapioca flour · 1 tsp xanthan gum · 1 packet dry yeast · 1 tbsp sugar · 1 tsp salt

1   First of all, pour the liquid ingredients to the bread baking machine. Mix all the dry ingredients in a bowl and place in the bread baking machine.

2   Bake the bread in the baking machine with a 3-hour white-bread program (usually program 1 or 2).

3   Depending on how well you can tolerate dairy products, you may be able to add 100–200 g of skimmed milk powder.

Bread with a long tradition...

Corn Bread

🕐 Baking time approx. 3 hours in a bread baking machine

200 mL of water · 100 mL of lactose-free milk · 1 tbsp vegetable oil · 200 g corn flour · 100 g potato starch · 200 g spelt flour · ½ tsp guar gum · 1 packet dry yeast · 1 tsp sugar · 1 sp salt

1   First of all, pour the liquid ingredients into the bread baking machine. Then add the dry ingredients.

2   Bake the bread in the baking machine with a white-bread program or a full-grain program of approx. 3 hours' baking time. Adjust the baking time according to the desired baking result.

Corn

Corn is gluten-free and originates from Mexico. In Mexico and the Southern states of the USA, corn is still regularly consumed in large quantities. Likely, Christopher Columbus brought corn from America to Europe.

The classic cornflakes and popcorn, which we like to eat in movie theaters, are made of corn, as is polenta, which is a popular side dish.

Corncob as a whole can be prepared in a number of ways. Seasoned with butter, salt and spices, it tastes perfect grilled, stewed or cooked. If you choose to cook corncobs, do not salt the water to prevent the corn kernels from becoming hard.

Season to taste ...

Cumin & Millet Bread

⌚ Baking time approx. 3 hours in a bread baking machine

300 mL of water · 230 g of millet flour · 70 g of potato starch · 1 tsp guar gum · 1 packet dry yeast · 30 g dry sour dough · 1 tsp caraway · 1 pinch of salt

1   Pour water into the bread baking machine. Then add the dry ingredients.

2   For baking, choose a standard or a white-bread program with a total time of approx. 3 hours. Adjust the baking time according to the baking result.

3   Give your creativity free reign with this bread. Try adding 1 tbsp of fresh thyme or 1 tbsp of sunflower seed instead of caraway.

Millet

Millet is one of the gluten-free cereals and was consumed a lot in Europe in the Middle Ages. With he arrival of corn and potatoes, however, millet started disappearing from the diet.

The recent comeback of millet is due to its many valuable ingredients and the various ways it can be used. It tastes well in sweets and as a side dish. Due to its relatively high fat content, it does not last as long as other cereals and should not be stored in large quantities.

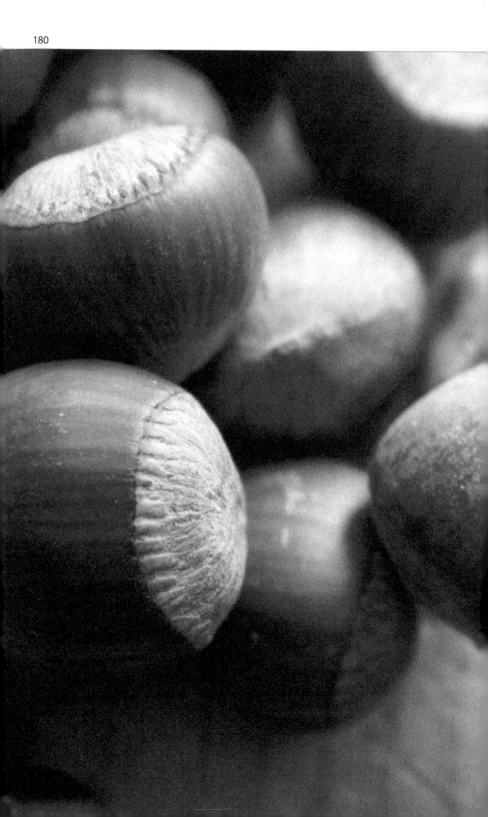

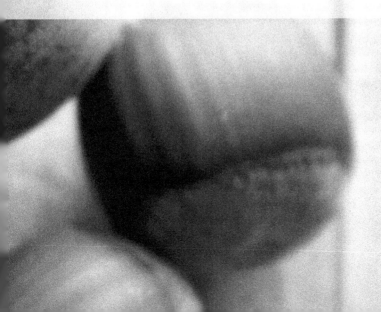

Appendix

Further Information

Academic or governmental organisations providing information on Irritable Bowel Syndrome (IBS):

International Foundation for Functional Gastrointestinal Disorders (IFFGD): https://www.aboutibs.org

Mayo Clinic, Rochester, Minnesota, USA:

https://www.mayoclinic.org/diseases-conditions/irritable-bowel-syndrome/symptoms-causes/syc-20360016

National Health Service, UK:

https://www.nhs.uk/conditions/irritable-bowel-syndrome-ibs/

Healthdirect, Government, Australia:

https://www.healthdirect.gov.au/irritable-bowel-syndrome-ibs

Charities and patient communities:

International Foundation for Functional Gastrointestinal Disorders (IFFGD), USA: https://www.iffgd.org/

IBS-Network, UK: https://www.theibsnetwork.org/

Betterhealth, Australia:

https://www.betterhealth.vic.gov.au/health/conditionsandtreatments/irritable-bowel-syndrome-ibs

Important scientific terms explained

Antibodies	Body's own proteins, formed during the immune reaction
Carbohydrates	Group of substances consisting of single or multiple sugars
Celiac disease	Autoimmune disease characterized by hypersensitivity to gluten
Crohn's Disease	Inflammatory bowel disease (chronic), affecting mostly the small intestine and colon
Disaccharides	Double sugars
Enzymes	Proteins that drive metabolic processes
Fermentation	Disintegration/Conversion of natural substances by microbial enzymes
Flatulence	Increased discharge of intestinal gases through the anus
FODMAP	Group of poorly digestible short-chain carbohydrates and polyols
Food additive designation	Numerical labeling of food additives (EXXX)
Fructans	Polysaccharides (multiple-unit sugars) that are composed of fructose molecules
Fructose	Fruit sugar
Fructose intolerance	Symptom-causing intolerance to fruit sugar
Galactans	Polysaccharides (multiple-unit sugars) composed of galactose molecules
Galactose	Simple sugar, also called „brain sugar"
Gliadins	Proteins contained in wheat
Glucose	Dextrose
Gluten	A composite of proteins stored in various grains
Gluten sensitivity	Sensitivity against gluten
Intestinal flora	Bacteria and other germs resident in the bowel
Inulin	Polysaccharide consisting of more than 100 fructose molecules
Irritable bowel syndrome	Functional intestinal disorder with digestive problems persisting over a longer period of time and impairing the quality of life
Lactase	Enzyme that cleaves milk sugar (lactose)
Lactose	Milk sugar

Lactose intolerance	Inability to easily digest lactose, a type of natural sugar found in milk and dairy products.
Monosaccharides	Simple sugars
Oligosaccharides	Carbohydrates consisting of 3-10 simple sugars
Polyols	Alcohols which are used in the food sector as sugar substitutes
Polysaccharides	Carbohydrates consisting of more than 10 simple sugars
Resistant starch	Starch that humans cannot digest
Retrograded starch	Starch that has become indigestible by heating and subsequent cooling
Saccharose	Table sugar
Sorbit/Sorbitol	Frequently used sugar substitute
Sugar alcohols	Sugar substitutes
Ulcerative colitis	Chronic inflammatory disease of the colon
Visceral hypersensitivity	Increased sensitivity to pain in the intestine
Wheat allergy	Genuine allergy to wheat ingredients
Wheat sensitivity	Wheat intolerance (previously also gluten sensitivity)

Recipes (alphabetically)

CPSIA information can be obtained
at www.ICGtesting.com
Printed in the USA
LVHW082237031119
636217LV00018B/871/P

9 781724 331809